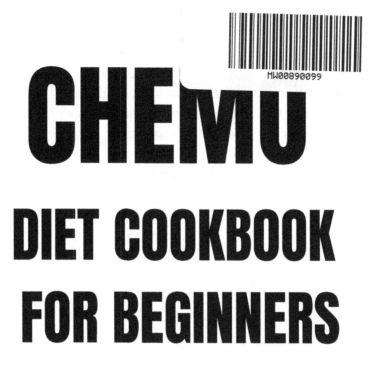

CHEMO
DIET COOKBOOK
FOR BEGINNERS

Easy, Nutritious Recipes for Wellness During and After Treatment

Kingsley Klopp

Table of Contents

Poultry Recipes

Fish & Seafood Recipes

Soup & Stew Recipes

Snacks & Desserts

10-WEEK MEAL PLAN

To show our appreciation for your purchase, we're delighted to offer you these special bonuses as a heartfelt thank you.

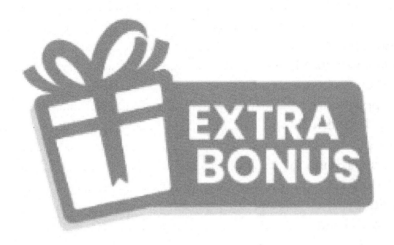

1. A Food Tracker Journal
2. Downloadable E-BOOK featuring full-color images of finished recipes

Important Note

We understand that this time may be overwhelming, and we're here to help you nourish your body and soul with comforting, nutritious meals.

It's important to note that individual dietary needs can vary greatly, especially during chemotherapy. What works well for one person may not suit another. As you explore the recipes in this cookbook, we encourage you to adjust them according to your own preferences and tolerances. Your healthcare team, including your doctor or a registered dietitian, can provide personalized guidance to ensure that your dietary choices align with your treatment plan.

Additionally, while we've provided nutritional information for each recipe, please understand that these values are approximate. The nutritional content can vary based on factors such as ingredient brands, portion sizes, and preparation methods. We recommend using this information as a general guide and adjusting as needed to meet your specific dietary requirements.

Cooking and eating during chemotherapy can be a way to regain a sense of control and comfort. This cookbook is more than just a collection of recipes; it's a companion on your journey to wellness. We've included practical tips, insights on managing side effects through diet, and encouragement to help you make each mealtime a positive experience.

Furthermore, If our cookbook has brought joy to your kitchen and table, we'd be thrilled to hear about your experiences in an Amazon review. On the flip side, if you stumble upon any hiccups while exploring our recipes, don't hesitate to get in touch at **kloppkingsley@gmail.com.** We're here to support your cooking journey every step of the way.

We hope that the **Chemo Diet Cookbook for Beginners** becomes a source of inspiration and support during this challenging time. May these recipes bring nourishment, enjoyment, and a moment of respite as you navigate through treatment.

Wishing you strength and good health,

Kingsley Klopp

Introduction

Hello there, and welcome! If you're holding this book, chances are you or someone you care about is facing the daunting challenge of chemotherapy. First off, let me say this: you're not alone. Whether you're just starting this journey or are well into it, navigating the world of chemotherapy can be overwhelming. But here's the good news: what you eat during this time can make a world of difference in how you feel and heal. In the midst of treatments and doctor visits, focusing on nutrition might seem like the last thing on your mind. Yet, what you put into your body can play a crucial role in supporting your strength, managing side effects, and boosting your overall well-being. That's where this cookbook comes in—it's your guide to delicious, nourishing meals tailored specifically for those undergoing chemotherapy.

Chemotherapy can affect your appetite, taste preferences, and digestion. It's not uncommon to experience changes in how foods taste or even in what you can tolerate eating. This cookbook is designed to help you navigate these challenges with recipes that are gentle on the stomach, packed with nutrients, and, most importantly, tasty enough to enjoy. What You'll Find Inside This isn't just any cookbook. It's a companion filled with easy-to-follow recipes that cater to beginners —whether you're new to cooking or simply new to cooking with your current dietary needs in mind. From comforting soups and stews to energizing smoothies and snacks, each recipe is crafted to be gentle on sensitive stomachs while delivering essential nutrients.

You don't need to be a chef to whip up these dishes. We've kept things straightforward with step-by-step instructions and readily available ingredients. Whether you're cooking for yourself or for someone dear to you, these recipes are designed to bring joy back to your kitchen and comfort to your table. Everyone's journey with chemotherapy is unique, and so are their dietary needs. Throughout this cookbook, you'll find tips on how to adapt recipes to fit your individual preferences and tolerances. Flexibility is key, and we encourage you to experiment with flavors and ingredients that work best for you.

While this cookbook provides practical guidance, it's essential to remember that your healthcare team is your primary resource. If you ever feel unsure about which foods to choose or how to manage specific symptoms through diet, don't hesitate to reach out to your doctor or a registered dietitian. They can offer personalized advice that complements your treatment plan. This book isn't just about meals; it's about nourishing your body and spirit during a challenging time. We've included insights on hydration, tips for boosting your appetite, and ideas for maintaining energy levels throughout your treatment. Because we believe that eating well is about more than just physical nourishment—it's about finding moments of comfort and joy amidst uncertainty.

So, are you ready to set out on a journey of healing and discovery through food? Let the **Chemo Diet Cookbook for Beginners** be your trusted companion, guiding you through flavorful recipes and empowering you to take control of your nutrition. Together, we'll make every meal a source of strength and comfort as you navigate this chapter of your life.

Part 1

The Basics of Chemotherapy and Nutrition

What is Chemotherapy?.

Chemotherapy is more than just a medical term; it is a journey, a battle, a glimmer of hope for those grappling with the often overwhelming diagnosis of cancer. For many, the word itself evokes a whirlwind of emotions—fear, uncertainty, courage, and resilience. But understanding chemotherapy, its purpose, and how it works can provide a sense of clarity and empowerment during a tumultuous time.

At its core, chemotherapy is a form of cancer treatment that uses powerful drugs to target and destroy rapidly dividing cancer cells. Unlike other treatments such as surgery or radiation, which are localized to specific areas, chemotherapy works systemically. This means it travels through the bloodstream, reaching cancer cells in almost every part of the body. For this reason, it is often the treatment of choice for cancers that have spread (metastasized) or are likely to do so.

The origins of chemotherapy date back to the early 20th century, when researchers discovered that certain chemical agents could shrink tumors in animals. This revelation sparked decades of research and development, leading to the diverse array of chemotherapy drugs available today. Each drug is meticulously designed to attack cancer cells at various stages of their life cycle, preventing them from growing and multiplying.

But what does this mean for those who undergo chemotherapy? It means embarking on a path filled with both challenges and triumphs. The process typically involves cycles of treatment, where periods of medication are followed by rest periods. These cycles are crucial, allowing the body to recover and build strength between treatments. Despite its lifesaving potential, chemotherapy is not without its hardships. The very nature of the treatment—targeting rapidly dividing cells—means that it can also affect healthy cells, particularly those that divide quickly, like those in the hair follicles, digestive tract, and bone marrow. This can lead to a range of side effects, including hair loss, nausea, fatigue, and a weakened immune system. Yet, it is important to remember that these side effects are often temporary and manageable. Medical teams work tirelessly to minimize discomfort and support patients through their treatment. Advances in medicine have led to the development of supportive care drugs that can alleviate many of these symptoms, making the journey a bit more bearable.

Beyond the physical aspects, chemotherapy also brings emotional and psychological challenges. The unpredictability of cancer and its treatment can be a source of immense stress and anxiety. Feelings of vulnerability and isolation are common as patients navigate the complexities of their new reality. However, this journey is rarely walked alone. Support from family, friends, healthcare providers, and fellow survivors can provide an invaluable network of strength and solidarity.

Chemotherapy is not just a battle against cancer; it is a testament to human resilience and the relentless pursuit of life. It is the embodiment of hope—a beacon that shines through the darkest moments, guiding patients towards recovery. The courage required to face chemotherapy is immense, and each step taken on this path is a victory in its own right. For those reading this, whether you are a patient, a loved one, or simply someone seeking to understand, know that chemotherapy is a powerful weapon in the fight against cancer. It is a complex, often grueling process, but one that holds the promise of healing and the possibility of a cancer-free future. Embrace the journey with hope and determination, for every story of survival begins with a single step forward.

The Role of Nutrition in Chemotherapy

When a person embarks on the daunting journey of chemotherapy, nutrition often becomes a powerful ally in their fight against cancer. The role of nutrition in chemotherapy is not just about maintaining strength and energy; it is about providing the body with the necessary tools to endure treatment, recover more effectively, and enhance overall well-being. This critical aspect of care can make a profound difference in a patient's experience and outcomes during one of the most challenging times in their life. Chemotherapy, by its very nature, is a rigorous process. It targets rapidly dividing cancer cells, but it also affects healthy cells, leading to a host of side effects such as nausea, fatigue, mouth sores, and changes in taste and appetite. These side effects can make eating feel like an insurmountable challenge. However, proper nutrition is essential for supporting the body's resilience and healing capabilities.

First and foremost, nutrition during chemotherapy is about sustaining energy. The body requires extra energy to repair itself and to combat the fatigue that often accompanies treatment. A well-balanced diet that includes adequate calories from a variety of sources—proteins, carbohydrates, and fats—is crucial. **Proteins**, in particular, are vital for repairing tissues and maintaining muscle mass. Lean meats, poultry, fish, eggs, dairy products, beans, and legumes are excellent sources of protein that can help keep the body strong. **Hydration** is another cornerstone of nutritional care during chemotherapy. Chemotherapy can cause dehydration due to vomiting, diarrhea, and decreased fluid intake. Drinking plenty of fluids, such as water, herbal teas, and broths, helps to keep the body hydrated, supports kidney function, and aids in the elimination of toxins from the body. **Fruits and vegetables** play an indispensable role in a chemotherapy diet. They are packed with vitamins, minerals, and antioxidants that help bolster the immune system and combat oxidative stress caused by treatment. However, it is important to ensure that they are washed thoroughly and prepared safely to reduce the risk of infections, as chemotherapy can weaken the immune system.

The emotional aspect of eating during chemotherapy should not be overlooked. Food can be a source of comfort and a semblance of normalcy amidst the chaos of treatment. However, it can also become a source of distress when side effects interfere with the ability to eat and enjoy meals. Finding ways to make eating more enjoyable, such as experimenting with different textures, flavors, and temperatures, can help. For instance, cold foods like smoothies or yogurt might be more tolerable than hot meals when dealing with mouth sores.

Managing side effects through nutrition is a key component of care. For nausea, small, frequent meals and bland, easy-to-digest foods like crackers, toast, and bananas can help. For those experiencing changes in taste, using herbs and spices to enhance the flavor of foods can make meals more palatable. If appetite is an issue, nutrient-dense snacks such as nuts, seeds, and avocados can provide necessary calories and nutrients in smaller portions. The support of a dietitian or nutritionist can be invaluable. These professionals can tailor dietary recommendations to individual needs, preferences, and tolerances, making the nutritional journey more personalized and manageable. They can also provide guidance on supplements if needed, though it is always best to get nutrients from food whenever possible.

Ultimately, the role of nutrition in chemotherapy is about more than just food; it is about nurturing the body and spirit. Good nutrition supports the physical demands of treatment, aids in recovery, and enhances quality of life. It is a vital part of the holistic care that cancer patients deserve, offering strength, comfort, and hope.

Common Side Effects of Chemotherapy and How Diet Can Help

1. **Nausea and Vomiting**: Nausea and vomiting are among the most common and distressing side effects of chemotherapy. They can make eating difficult and can lead to dehydration and nutritional deficiencies.

How Diet Can Help:

- Small, Frequent Meals: Eating smaller, more frequent meals rather than three large ones can help prevent an empty stomach, which can exacerbate nausea.
- Bland Foods: Bland, easy-to-digest foods like crackers, toast, and rice are often better tolerated.
- Ginger and Peppermint: Natural remedies like ginger tea or peppermint can help soothe the stomach.
- Hydration: Sipping on clear fluids like water, broth, and herbal teas can help maintain hydration and prevent vomiting.

2. **Fatigue:** Chemotherapy-induced fatigue is a persistent tiredness that can affect daily activities and overall energy levels.

How Diet Can Help:

- Balanced Diet: Eating a well-balanced diet rich in fruits, vegetables, lean proteins, and whole grains provides the body with essential nutrients and energy.
- Iron-Rich Foods: Consuming iron-rich foods like spinach, beans, and red meat can help combat anemia, a common cause of fatigue.
- Hydration: Staying hydrated helps maintain energy levels and prevent fatigue.

3. **Loss of Appetite**: Many patients experience a reduced appetite during chemotherapy, which can lead to unintended weight loss and malnutrition.

How Diet Can Help:

- Nutrient-Dense Foods: Focus on nutrient-dense foods that provide more calories and nutrients in smaller portions, such as nuts, seeds, avocados, and smoothies.
- Meal Timing: Eating when feeling most hungry, which might be in the morning for some, can help maximize food intake.
- Caloric Supplements: In some cases, high-calorie nutritional supplements can be beneficial.

4. **Mouth Sores (Mucositis):** Chemotherapy can cause painful sores in the mouth and throat, making eating difficult and uncomfortable.

How Diet Can Help:
- Soft Foods: Soft, soothing foods like yogurt, mashed potatoes, and smoothies are easier to eat and less likely to irritate sores.
- Avoid Irritants: Avoiding spicy, acidic, and rough-textured foods can prevent further irritation.
- Hydration: Drinking plenty of fluids can help keep the mouth moist and reduce discomfort.

5. Changes in Taste and Smell: Chemotherapy can alter taste and smell, making foods taste bland, metallic, or unpleasant.

How Diet Can Help:
- Experiment with Flavors: Using herbs, spices, and marinades can enhance the flavor of foods.
- Cold Foods: Cold foods, such as smoothies and chilled soups, might be more palatable than hot ones.
- Oral Hygiene: Good oral hygiene, including rinsing the mouth before meals, can help improve taste perception.

6. Diarrhea: Diarrhea can lead to dehydration and nutrient loss, posing significant health risks if not managed properly.

How Diet Can Help:
- Low-Fiber Foods: Consuming low-fiber foods like bananas, rice, applesauce, and toast can help reduce diarrhea.
- Hydration: Drinking plenty of fluids with electrolytes, such as oral rehydration solutions, helps maintain hydration.
- Small, Frequent Meals: Smaller, more frequent meals can be easier on the digestive system.

7. Constipation: Conversely, some chemotherapy treatments can cause constipation, leading to discomfort and bloating.

How Diet Can Help:
- High-Fiber Foods: Increasing intake of high-fiber foods such as fruits, vegetables, whole grains, and legumes can help promote regular bowel movements.
- Hydration: Drinking plenty of water aids in digestion and helps prevent constipation.
- Physical Activity: Light physical activity, as tolerated, can also help stimulate bowel movements.

Hence, while chemotherapy presents numerous side effects, diet and nutrition can significantly mitigate these challenges. By carefully selecting foods that soothe, nourish, and sustain, patients can better manage the physical toll of treatment. The support of healthcare professionals, including dietitians, can further tailor dietary approaches to individual needs, enhancing the therapeutic journey with strength and hope. Through mindful nutrition, the path through chemotherapy can become more manageable, promoting healing and improving quality of life.

Key Nutritional Needs During Chemotherapy

1. Caloric Intake: Maintaining Energy Levels Chemotherapy increases the body's energy demands, as it works to repair tissues and fight cancer. Maintaining adequate caloric intake is crucial to prevent weight loss and muscle wasting.

- Nutrient-Dense Foods: Focus on foods that provide high calories and essential nutrients in small portions, such as nuts, seeds, avocados, whole grains, and healthy oils.
- Frequent Meals: Eating small, frequent meals throughout the day can help sustain energy levels and make it easier to meet caloric needs, especially if appetite is reduced.

2. Protein: Building and Repairing Tissues Protein is vital for repairing tissues, maintaining muscle mass, and supporting immune function. Chemotherapy can lead to muscle wasting, making protein intake even more critical.

- Lean Proteins: Include sources of lean protein such as poultry, fish, eggs, low-fat dairy products, beans, and legumes.
- Protein Supplements: If food intake is insufficient, protein shakes or supplements can help meet daily protein requirements.

3. Hydration: Maintaining Fluid Balance Staying hydrated is essential during chemotherapy, as treatment can cause dehydration due to side effects like vomiting and diarrhea.

- Fluids: Drink plenty of fluids, such as water, herbal teas, clear broths, and electrolyte solutions.
- Hydrating Foods: Incorporate foods with high water content, like fruits (watermelon, oranges) and vegetables (cucumbers, celery), to boost hydration.

4. Vitamins and Minerals: Supporting Immune Function and Healing Vitamins and minerals are crucial for overall health, immune function, and healing. Chemotherapy can deplete certain nutrients, making it essential to replenish them through diet.

- Fruits and Vegetables: Aim for a variety of colorful fruits and vegetables to ensure a broad spectrum of vitamins and minerals.
- Whole Grains and Legumes: These are excellent sources of B vitamins, iron, and magnesium.
- Supplements: Consult with a healthcare provider before taking any supplements, as some may interact with chemotherapy.

5. Fats: Providing Energy and Supporting Cell Function Healthy fats are a concentrated source of energy and play a role in cell function and the absorption of fat-soluble vitamins (A, D, E, and K).

- Healthy Fats: Include sources of healthy fats such as olive oil, avocados, nuts, seeds, and fatty fish (salmon, mackerel).

6. Fiber: Supporting Digestive Health Chemotherapy can affect the digestive system, causing constipation or diarrhea. Fiber plays a key role in maintaining digestive health and regular bowel movements.

- Soluble Fiber: For diarrhea, soluble fiber from foods like oats, bananas, and apples can help solidify stools.
- Insoluble Fiber: For constipation, insoluble fiber from whole grains, vegetables, and legumes can help promote regularity.
- Fluid Intake: Ensure adequate fluid intake when increasing fiber to prevent constipation.

7. Special Considerations: Managing Side Effects Through Diet Diet can be adjusted to manage specific side effects of chemotherapy.

- Nausea and Vomiting: Eat bland, easy-to-digest foods like crackers, toast, and rice. Ginger tea or ginger candies can help soothe nausea.
- Mouth Sores: Opt for soft, non-acidic foods like yogurt, mashed potatoes, and smoothies. Avoid spicy, salty, and rough-textured foods.
- Taste Changes: Enhance the flavor of foods with herbs, spices, and marinades. Cold foods might be more palatable if taste changes are severe.
- Fatigue: Eat nutrient-dense foods that provide sustained energy, such as whole grains, lean proteins, and healthy fats. Avoid sugary snacks that can cause energy crashes.

8. Individualized Nutrition Plans: Personalizing Care Each patient's nutritional needs during chemotherapy are unique, influenced by the type of cancer, treatment plan, side effects, and individual preferences.

- Dietitian Support: Working with a registered dietitian can help tailor a nutrition plan to meet specific needs and preferences, ensuring optimal support throughout treatment.
- Flexibility: Be flexible and adjust the diet as needed to accommodate changing symptoms and preferences.

Foods to Include

1. Lean Proteins: Building and Repairing Tissues Protein is essential for repairing tissues, maintaining muscle mass, and supporting the immune system. During chemotherapy, the body requires more protein to help recover from the damage caused by treatment.

- Poultry and Fish: Chicken, turkey, and fish like salmon and cod are excellent sources of lean protein.
- Eggs: Packed with protein and easy to digest, eggs are a versatile addition to the diet.
- Low-Fat Dairy: Options like yogurt, milk, and cottage cheese provide protein and are often fortified with additional nutrients.
- Legumes: Beans, lentils, and chickpeas are plant-based protein sources that also provide fiber and other essential nutrients.
- Tofu and Tempeh: These soy products are great for those who prefer plant-based proteins and can be incorporated into a variety of dishes.

2. Whole Grains: Sustaining Energy Levels Whole grains provide complex carbohydrates that offer sustained energy, along with fiber, vitamins, and minerals.

- Oats: A comforting and nutritious option for breakfast or snacks.
- Brown Rice and Quinoa: These grains are high in fiber and can be used as a base for many meals.
- Whole Wheat Bread and Pasta: These options are more nutritious than their refined counterparts and help maintain energy levels throughout the day.
- Barley and Bulgur: These grains add variety and texture to meals while providing essential nutrients.

3. Fruits and Vegetables: Boosting Immune Function and Reducing Inflammation Fruits and vegetables are rich in vitamins, minerals, and antioxidants that help support the immune system and reduce inflammation.

- Berries: Blueberries, strawberries, and raspberries are high in antioxidants and can be enjoyed fresh or in smoothies.
- Leafy Greens: Spinach, kale, and Swiss chard are nutrient-dense and can be added to salads, soups, or smoothies.
- Cruciferous Vegetables: Broccoli, cauliflower, and Brussels sprouts contain compounds that support detoxification and immune health, but they should be cooked and consumed in moderation if they cause digestive issues.
- Citrus Fruits: Oranges, grapefruits, and lemons are high in vitamin C, which supports the immune system and aids in iron absorption.
- Colorful Vegetables: Bell peppers, carrots, and sweet potatoes provide a range of vitamins and minerals essential for overall health.

4. Healthy Fats: Supporting Cell Function and Absorption of Nutrients Healthy fats are a concentrated source of energy and help absorb fat-soluble vitamins (A, D, E, and K).

- Avocados: Rich in healthy monounsaturated fats and fiber, avocados are a versatile addition to meals.
- Nuts and Seeds: Almonds, walnuts, chia seeds, and flaxseeds provide healthy fats, protein, and fiber.
- Olive Oil: A staple of the Mediterranean diet, olive oil is high in monounsaturated fats and can be used in cooking or as a salad dressing.
- Fatty Fish: Salmon, mackerel, and sardines are excellent sources of omega-3 fatty acids, which have anti-inflammatory properties.

5. Hydrating Foods: Maintaining Fluid Balance Staying hydrated is crucial during chemotherapy, as treatment can lead to dehydration due to side effects like vomiting and diarrhea.

- Water-Rich Fruits and Vegetables: Cucumbers, watermelon, and celery help maintain hydration levels.
- Broths and Soups: These provide fluids and electrolytes while being easy to digest.
- Herbal Teas: Ginger, peppermint, and chamomile teas can be soothing and help with nausea.

6. Fermented Foods: Supporting Digestive Health Fermented foods contain probiotics that support gut health, which can be disrupted by chemotherapy.

- Yogurt and Kefir: These dairy products are rich in probiotics and can be consumed on their own or added to smoothies.
- Sauerkraut and Kimchi: Fermented vegetables that provide beneficial bacteria and add a tangy flavor to meals.
- Miso and Tempeh: These soy-based products are not only sources of protein but also contain probiotics.

7. High-Calorie, Nutrient-Dense Snacks: Preventing Weight Loss Maintaining weight during chemotherapy can be challenging due to loss of appetite and increased energy needs. Including high-calorie, nutrient-dense snacks can help.

- Nut Butters: Peanut butter, almond butter, and other nut butters are calorie-dense and can be added to smoothies, spread on toast, or eaten with fruits.
- Trail Mix: A mix of nuts, seeds, and dried fruits provides calories, protein, and healthy fats.
- Smoothies: Blended drinks with fruits, vegetables, protein powder, and healthy fats can be a convenient way to intake nutrients and calories.

8. Comfort Foods: Providing Emotional and Physical Comfort Comfort foods can help soothe the body and mind, especially when dealing with the stress and discomfort of chemotherapy.

- Warm, Soft Foods: Mashed potatoes, oatmeal, and soups can be easier to eat and digest, providing both physical and emotional comfort.
- Familiar Favorites: Sometimes, eating favorite foods, even in small amounts, can help maintain a sense of normalcy and enjoyment in eating.

Foods to Avoid

1. **Processed and Sugary Foods**: Reducing Inflammation and Maintaining Energy Levels Processed and sugary foods can lead to inflammation, spikes in blood sugar levels, and energy crashes. They also lack essential nutrients that the body needs during chemotherapy.

- Sugary Snacks and Desserts: Items like candy, cookies, cakes, and pastries should be limited. These foods provide empty calories without nutritional benefits.
- Processed Foods: Foods such as packaged snacks, fast food, and ready-made meals often contain high levels of unhealthy fats, sodium, and preservatives.
- Sugary Beverages: Sodas, energy drinks, and other sugary beverages can lead to rapid changes in blood sugar levels, contributing to fatigue and other side effects.

2. **High-Fat and Fried Foods**: Managing Digestive Discomfort High-fat and fried foods can be difficult to digest and may exacerbate side effects like nausea, vomiting, and diarrhea.

- Fried Foods: Items like fried chicken, French fries, and other deep-fried foods should be avoided as they can cause indigestion and discomfort.
- High-Fat Meats: Fatty cuts of meat, bacon, sausage, and other high-fat meats can be hard to digest and may contribute to feelings of nausea.
- Rich Desserts: Creamy desserts, ice cream, and foods high in saturated fats should be limited.

3. **Spicy and Acidic Foods**: Preventing Irritation of the Digestive Tract Spicy and acidic foods can irritate the mouth, throat, and stomach, which may already be sensitive due to chemotherapy.

- Spicy Foods: Hot peppers, spicy sauces, and heavily spiced dishes can cause discomfort and exacerbate mouth sores.
- Acidic Foods: Citrus fruits (lemons, oranges, grapefruits), tomatoes, and vinegar-based foods can irritate the mouth and digestive tract.
- Carbonated Beverages: Sodas and sparkling water can increase acidity and cause bloating or discomfort.

4. Raw or Undercooked Foods: Minimizing Risk of Infection Chemotherapy can weaken the immune system, making patients more susceptible to infections. Consuming raw or undercooked foods can increase the risk of foodborne illnesses.

- Raw Meat and Fish: Avoid sushi, sashimi, and undercooked meats to reduce the risk of bacterial contamination.
- Raw Eggs: Foods containing raw eggs, like certain homemade dressings, mayonnaise, and cookie dough, should be avoided.
- Unpasteurized Dairy: Unpasteurized milk, cheese, and other dairy products can harbor harmful bacteria.

5. High-Fiber Foods: Managing Digestive Issues While fiber is generally beneficial, high-fiber foods can worsen certain digestive side effects like diarrhea.

- Cruciferous Vegetables: Broccoli, cauliflower, and Brussels sprouts can cause gas and bloating. These should be cooked thoroughly and consumed in moderation if they are well tolerated.
- Whole Grains: Foods like brown rice, whole wheat bread, and high-fiber cereals may be too harsh on a sensitive digestive system during chemotherapy.
- Legumes: Beans, lentils, and chickpeas can cause gas and discomfort.

6. Alcohol: Avoiding Negative Interactions with Treatment Alcohol can interfere with the effectiveness of chemotherapy and exacerbate its side effects.

- Alcoholic Beverages: Wine, beer, and spirits can irritate the stomach lining, contribute to dehydration, and negatively interact with medications.

7. Caffeinated Beverages: Managing Dehydration and Anxiety Excessive caffeine can lead to dehydration and exacerbate anxiety or sleep disturbances.

- Coffee and Energy Drinks: High-caffeine drinks should be limited to prevent dehydration and jitteriness.
- Certain Teas and Sodas: Some teas and sodas also contain caffeine and should be consumed in moderation.

8. Artificial Additives and Preservatives: Reducing Chemical Exposure Artificial additives and preservatives can introduce unnecessary chemicals into the body, which is already under stress from chemotherapy.

- Artificial Sweeteners: Aspartame, saccharin, and sucralose may cause gastrointestinal upset in some people.
- Preservative-Laden Foods: Processed meats, packaged snacks, and other foods high in preservatives should be avoided.

9. Very Hot or Cold Foods: Preventing Sensitivity Issues Extreme temperatures can be uncomfortable for those experiencing mouth sores or sensitivity.

- Piping Hot Foods and Beverages: Foods that are too hot can further irritate the mouth and throat.
- Ice-Cold Foods and Beverages: Extremely cold items can cause discomfort in sensitive areas of the mouth.

Further Clarification

We cannot emphasize this enough: the impact of chemotherapy on individuals can vary greatly. What works harmoniously for one person may induce unexpected reactions in another. As such, it's crucial to recognize that the recipes featured in this cookbook are crafted specifically for those undergoing or who have undergone chemotherapy. Each individual's body responds uniquely to treatments and dietary adjustments. Chemotherapy can alter taste preferences, digestion, and overall tolerance to certain foods. While we have curated these recipes with care and consideration, we urge you to remain attentive to your body's signals. If you find that a particular ingredient triggers discomfort or intolerance, we encourage you to substitute or adjust it accordingly. Furthermore, consulting with your healthcare team—comprising oncologists, dietitians, and other specialists—is vital. They can provide personalized advice tailored to your specific medical needs and treatment plan. Your health and well-being are our utmost priority, and we want your experience with this cookbook to be both supportive and empowering. It's also important to note that the nutritional information provided alongside each recipe is intended as a general guideline. Variations in ingredients, portion sizes, and preparation methods can affect nutritional values. Therefore, we recommend using this information as a reference point while adapting recipes to suit your dietary requirements.

Above all, we understand the emotional and physical challenges that come with chemotherapy. Our goal is to offer not only nourishing meal options but also a sense of comfort and reassurance during this time. We hope that the **"Chemo Diet Cookbook for Beginners"** serves as a valuable resource in your journey towards wellness.

Breakfast Recipes

1. Barley Porridge with Dates and Almonds

Ingredients:

- 1 cup pearl barley
- 4 cups water
- 1 cup almond milk (unsweetened)
- 1/4 cup chopped dates
- 1/4 cup sliced almonds
- 1 tablespoon honey
- 1 teaspoon vanilla extract
- 1/2 teaspoon ground cinnamon

Instructions:

1. Rinse the pearl barley under cold water.
2. In a large pot, combine the barley and water. Bring to a boil over medium heat.
3. Reduce the heat to low, cover, and simmer for 45 minutes, or until the barley is tender.
4. Drain any excess water and return the barley to the pot.
5. Stir in the almond milk, dates, honey, vanilla extract, and ground cinnamon.
6. Cook over low heat for an additional 10 minutes, stirring occasionally, until the porridge is creamy and heated through.
7. Serve hot, topped with sliced almonds.

Nutrition Info per Serving:

- Calories: 280
- Protein: 7g
- Carbohydrates: 50g
- Fat: 6g
- Fiber: 8g
- Sugar: 14g

Number of Serves: 4
Cooking Time: 55 minutes

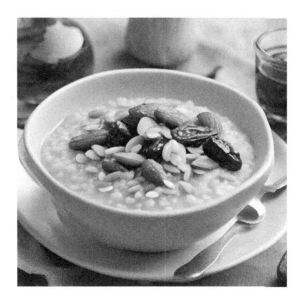

2. Peach and Ginger Compote

Ingredients:

- 4 ripe peaches, peeled, pitted, and sliced
- 1/4 cup water
- 1 tablespoon fresh ginger, grated
- 2 tablespoons honey
- 1 teaspoon vanilla extract

Instructions:

1. In a medium saucepan, combine the peaches, water, and grated ginger.
2. Cook over medium heat, stirring occasionally, until the peaches begin to soften, about 10 minutes.
3. Stir in the honey and vanilla extract.
4. Continue to cook for an additional 5 minutes, or until the peaches are tender and the compote has thickened slightly.
5. Remove from heat and let cool slightly before serving.

Nutrition Info per Serving:

- Calories: 100
- Protein: 1g
- Carbohydrates: 26g
- Fat: 0g
- Fiber: 2g
- Sugar: 23g

Number of Serves: 4
Cooking Time: 15 minutes

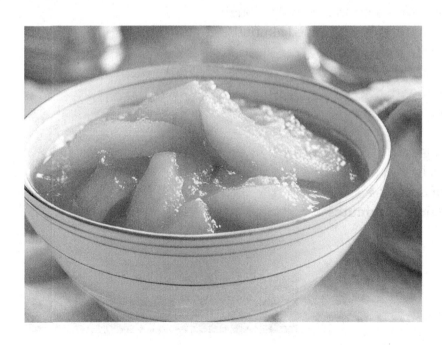

3. Raspberry and Walnut Oatmeal

Ingredients:

- 1 cup rolled oats
- 2 cups water
- 1 cup almond milk (unsweetened)
- 1 cup fresh raspberries
- 1/4 cup chopped walnuts
- 1 tablespoon honey
- 1 teaspoon vanilla extract
- 1/2 teaspoon ground cinnamon

Instructions:

1. In a medium saucepan, combine the rolled oats, water, and almond milk. Bring to a boil over medium heat.
2. Reduce heat to low and simmer for 5-7 minutes, or until the oats are tender and the mixture is creamy.
3. Stir in the honey, vanilla extract, and ground cinnamon.
4. Serve hot, topped with fresh raspberries and chopped walnuts.

Nutrition Info per Serving:

- Calories: 230
- Protein: 6g
- Carbohydrates: 34g
- Fat: 10g
- Fiber: 7g
- Sugar: 10g

Number of Serves: 4
Cooking Time: 10 minutes

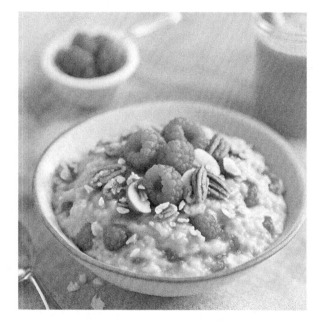

4. Egg Custard

Ingredients:

- 4 large eggs
- 2 cups almond milk (unsweetened)
- 1/4 cup honey
- 1 teaspoon vanilla extract
- 1/2 teaspoon ground nutmeg

Instructions:

1. Preheat the oven to 350°F (175°C).
2. In a medium bowl, whisk together the eggs, almond milk, honey, and vanilla extract until well combined.
3. Pour the mixture into individual custard cups or ramekins.
4. Place the custard cups in a baking dish and add enough hot water to the baking dish to come halfway up the sides of the cups.
5. Sprinkle the tops with ground nutmeg.
6. Bake for 30-35 minutes, or until the custards are set and a knife inserted into the center comes out clean.
7. Remove from the oven and let cool slightly before serving.

Nutrition Info per Serving:

- Calories: 140
- Protein: 6g
- Carbohydrates: 19g
- Fat: 5g
- Fiber: 0g
- Sugar: 18g

Number of Serves: 4
Cooking Time: 35 minutes

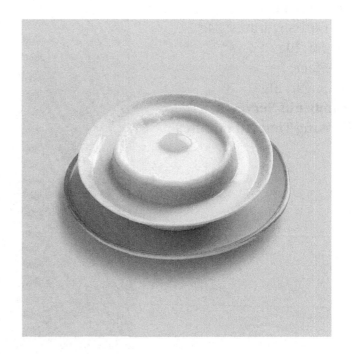

5. Kefir with Honey and Almonds

Ingredients:

- 2 cups plain kefir
- 2 tablespoons honey
- 1/4 cup sliced almonds
- 1 teaspoon vanilla extract

Instructions:

1. In a medium bowl, whisk together the plain kefir, honey, and vanilla extract until well combined.
2. Pour the kefir mixture into serving glasses or bowls.
3. Top each serving with sliced almonds.
4. Serve immediately.

Nutrition Info per Serving:

- Calories: 160
- Protein: 6g
- Carbohydrates: 20g
- Fat: 7g
- Fiber: 2g
- Sugar: 16g

Number of Serves: 4
Cooking Time: 5 minutes

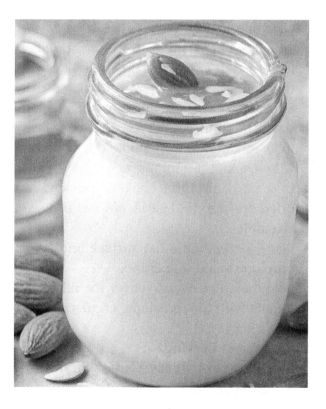

6. Spinach and Cheese Stuffed Crepes

Ingredients:

- **For the crepes:**
  - 1 cup whole wheat flour
  - 2 large eggs
  - 1 1/2 cups almond milk (unsweetened)
  - 1 tablespoon olive oil
  - 1 teaspoon vanilla extract
- For the filling:
  - 2 cups fresh spinach, chopped
  - 1 cup ricotta cheese
  - 1/2 cup shredded mozzarella cheese
  - 1 teaspoon dried oregano
  - 1 teaspoon garlic powder

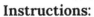

Instructions:

1. **To make the crepes:**
   - In a large bowl, whisk together the whole wheat flour, eggs, almond milk, olive oil, and vanilla extract until smooth.
   - Heat a non-stick skillet over medium heat and lightly grease it with a little olive oil.
   - Pour 1/4 cup of the batter into the skillet and swirl to spread it evenly. Cook for about 1-2 minutes on each side, until the crepe is golden and cooked through.
   - Repeat with the remaining batter, stacking the cooked crepes on a plate.
2. **To make the filling:**
   - In a medium skillet, cook the chopped spinach over medium heat until wilted, about 3-4 minutes.
   - In a bowl, mix the cooked spinach, ricotta cheese, shredded mozzarella, dried oregano, and garlic powder until well combined.
3. **To assemble:**
   - Place a crepe on a flat surface and spoon about 2 tablespoons of the filling onto one half of the crepe.
   - Fold the crepe over to cover the filling, and then fold again to form a triangle.
   - Repeat with the remaining crepes and filling.
   - Serve warm.

Nutrition Info per Serving:

- Calories: 230 Protein: 12g Carbohydrates: 20g Fat: 12g
- Fiber: 2g Sugar: 3g

Number of Serves: 6

Cooking Time: 30 minutes

7. Butternut Squash Soup

Ingredients:

- 1 medium butternut squash, peeled, seeded, and cubed
- 1 medium onion, chopped
- 2 cloves garlic, minced
- 4 cups low-sodium vegetable broth
- 1 cup almond milk (unsweetened)
- 1 teaspoon ground ginger
- 1 teaspoon ground cinnamon
- 1 tablespoon olive oil

Instructions:

1. In a large pot, heat the olive oil over medium heat. Add the chopped onion and garlic, and cook until softened, about 5 minutes.
2. Add the cubed butternut squash and ground ginger, and cook for another 5 minutes, stirring occasionally.
3. Pour in the vegetable broth and bring to a boil. Reduce the heat and simmer until the squash is tender, about 20 minutes.
4. Use an immersion blender to puree the soup until smooth. Alternatively, transfer the soup to a blender in batches and blend until smooth.
5. Stir in the almond milk and ground cinnamon. Heat through, but do not boil.
6. Serve warm.

Nutrition Info per Serving:

- Calories: 120
- Protein: 2g
- Carbohydrates: 26g
- Fat: 3g
- Fiber: 4g
- Sugar: 7g

Number of Serves: 4
Cooking Time: 30 minutes

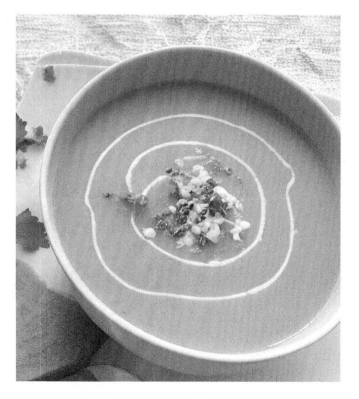

8. Herbed Scrambled Tofu

Ingredients:

- 1 block firm tofu, drained and crumbled
- 1 small onion, finely chopped
- 1 bell pepper, finely chopped
- 1 cup fresh spinach, chopped
- 2 tablespoons nutritional yeast
- 1 teaspoon turmeric powder
- 1 teaspoon dried thyme
- 1 tablespoon olive oil

Instructions:

1. In a large skillet, heat the olive oil over medium heat. Add the chopped onion and bell pepper, and cook until softened, about 5 minutes.
2. Add the crumbled tofu to the skillet, along with the turmeric powder and dried thyme. Cook, stirring occasionally, until the tofu is heated through and well combined with the spices, about 5-7 minutes.
3. Stir in the chopped spinach and nutritional yeast, and cook until the spinach is wilted, about 2 minutes.
4. Serve warm.

Nutrition Info per Serving:

- Calories: 180
- Protein: 12g
- Carbohydrates: 8g
- Fat: 12g
- Fiber: 3g
- Sugar: 2g

Number of Serves: 4
Cooking Time: 15 minutes

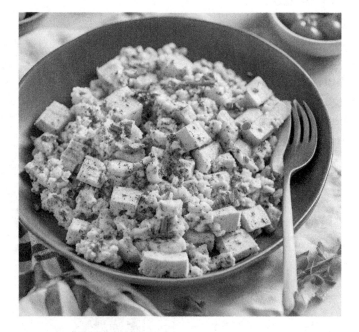

9. Pancakes with Ricotta and Orange Zest

Ingredients:

- 1 cup whole wheat flour
- 1 tablespoon baking powder
- 1 cup almond milk (unsweetened)
- 1/2 cup ricotta cheese
- 2 large eggs
- 1 tablespoon honey
- 1 teaspoon vanilla extract
- 1 tablespoon orange zest

Instructions:

1. In a large bowl, whisk together the whole wheat flour and baking powder.
2. In another bowl, whisk together the almond milk, ricotta cheese, eggs, honey, and vanilla extract until smooth.
3. Pour the wet ingredients into the dry ingredients and mix until just combined. Stir in the orange zest.
4. Heat a non-stick skillet over medium heat and lightly grease it with a little olive oil.
5. Pour 1/4 cup of the batter into the skillet for each pancake. Cook for about 2-3 minutes on each side, until golden and cooked through.
6. Serve warm with additional honey or fresh fruit if desired.

Nutrition Info per Serving:

- Calories: 200
- Protein: 8g
- Carbohydrates: 28g
- Fat: 6g
- Fiber: 3g
- Sugar: 8g

Number of Serves: 4
Cooking Time: 20 minutes

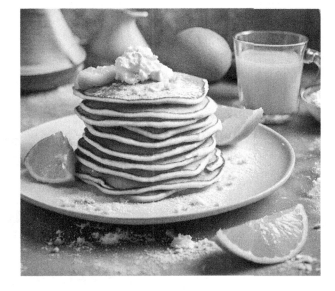

10. Vegetable Omelette

Ingredients:

- 4 large eggs
- 1/2 cup almond milk (unsweetened)
- 1 small onion, finely chopped
- 1 small bell pepper, finely chopped
- 1 small tomato, diced
- 1 cup fresh spinach, chopped
- 1/4 cup shredded mozzarella cheese
- 1 tablespoon olive oil
- 1 teaspoon dried basil

Instructions:

1. In a bowl, whisk together the eggs and almond milk until well combined.
2. In a large non-stick skillet, heat the olive oil over medium heat. Add the chopped onion and bell pepper, and cook until softened, about 5 minutes.
3. Add the diced tomato and chopped spinach to the skillet, and cook until the spinach is wilted, about 2 minutes.
4. Pour the egg mixture over the vegetables and cook without stirring until the eggs begin to set, about 3 minutes.
5. Sprinkle the shredded mozzarella cheese and dried basil over the omelette.
6. Fold the omelette in half and continue cooking until the eggs are fully set and the cheese is melted, about 2 minutes.
7. Serve warm.

Nutrition Info per Serving:

- Calories: 220
- Protein: 14g
- Carbohydrates: 7g
- Fat: 15g
- Fiber: 2g
- Sugar: 4g

Number of Serves: 2
Cooking Time: 15 minutes

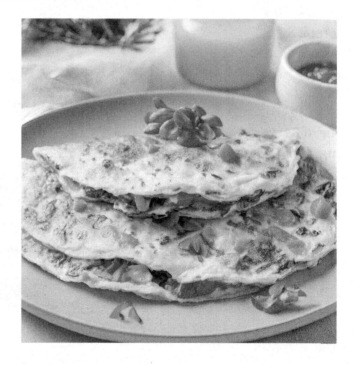

11. Soft French Toast with Apple Compote

Ingredients:

- **For the French Toast:**
  - 4 slices whole wheat bread
  - 2 large eggs
  - 1 cup almond milk (unsweetened)
  - 1 tablespoon honey
  - 1 teaspoon vanilla extract
  - 1/2 teaspoon ground cinnamon
  - 1 tablespoon olive oil
- For the Apple Compote:
  - 2 medium apples, peeled, cored, and chopped
  - 1/4 cup water
  - 1 tablespoon honey
  - 1 teaspoon ground cinnamon
  - 1 teaspoon vanilla extract

Instructions:

1. **To make the Apple Compote:**
   - In a medium saucepan, combine the chopped apples, water, honey, cinnamon, and vanilla extract.
   - Cook over medium heat, stirring occasionally, until the apples are soft and the mixture has thickened, about 10 minutes. Set aside.
2. **To make the French Toast:**
   - In a shallow bowl, whisk together the eggs, almond milk, honey, vanilla extract, and ground cinnamon.
   - Heat the olive oil in a large non-stick skillet over medium heat.
   - Dip each slice of bread into the egg mixture, ensuring both sides are well-coated.
   - Cook the bread slices in the skillet until golden brown, about 2-3 minutes per side.
   - Serve the French toast topped with the apple compote.

Nutrition Info per Serving:

- Calories: 280
- Protein: 9g
- Carbohydrates: 45g
- Fat: 8g
- Fiber: 6g
- Sugar: 20g

Number of Serves: 2
Cooking Time: 20 minutes

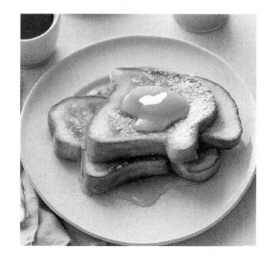

12. Chia Pudding with Kiwi

Ingredients:

- 1/4 cup chia seeds
- 1 cup almond milk (unsweetened)
- 1 tablespoon honey
- 1 teaspoon vanilla extract
- 2 kiwis, peeled and sliced

Instructions:

1. In a medium bowl, whisk together the chia seeds, almond milk, honey, and vanilla extract.
2. Cover and refrigerate for at least 4 hours, or overnight, until the mixture has thickened to a pudding-like consistency.
3. Stir the pudding before serving.
4. Top with sliced kiwi and serve chilled.

Nutrition Info per Serving:

- Calories: 200
- Protein: 6g
- Carbohydrates: 30g
- Fat: 8g
- Fiber: 9g
- Sugar: 12g

Number of Serves: 2

Cooking Time: 10 minutes (plus refrigeration time)

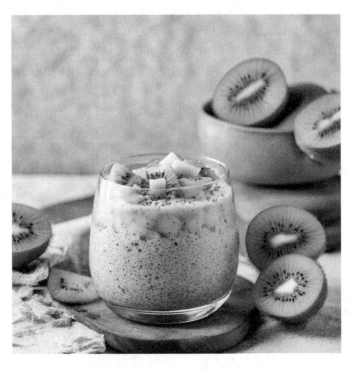

13. Baked Sweet Potatoes with Yogurt and Chives

Ingredients:

- 2 medium sweet potatoes
- 1/2 cup plain Greek yogurt
- 2 tablespoons chopped fresh chives
- 1 tablespoon olive oil

Instructions:

1. Preheat the oven to 400°F (200°C).
2. Wash the sweet potatoes and pierce them several times with a fork.
3. Rub the sweet potatoes with olive oil and place them on a baking sheet.
4. Bake for 45-50 minutes, or until tender.
5. Cut the sweet potatoes in half lengthwise and fluff the insides with a fork.
6. Top each half with a dollop of Greek yogurt and sprinkle with chopped chives.
7. Serve warm.

Nutrition Info per Serving:

- Calories: 180
- Protein: 5g
- Carbohydrates: 32g
- Fat: 5g
- Fiber: 5g
- Sugar: 7g

Number of Serves: 2

Cooking Time: 50 minutes

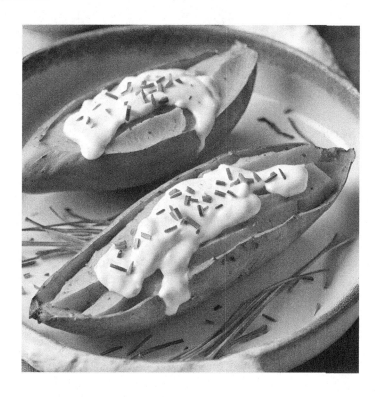

14. Sweet Corn Cakes

Ingredients:

- 1 cup cornmeal
- 1/2 cup whole wheat flour
- 1 teaspoon baking powder
- 1 cup almond milk (unsweetened)
- 1 cup fresh or frozen corn kernels
- 2 large eggs
- 1 tablespoon honey
- 1 teaspoon vanilla extract
- 1 tablespoon olive oil

Instructions:

1. In a large bowl, mix together the cornmeal, whole wheat flour, and baking powder.
2. In another bowl, whisk together the almond milk, eggs, honey, and vanilla extract.
3. Pour the wet ingredients into the dry ingredients and mix until just combined. Stir in the corn kernels.
4. Heat the olive oil in a large non-stick skillet over medium heat.
5. Pour 1/4 cup of the batter into the skillet for each corn cake. Cook for 2-3 minutes on each side, until golden and cooked through.
6. Serve warm.

Nutrition Info per Serving:

- Calories: 220
- Protein: 7g
- Carbohydrates: 32g
- Fat: 7g
- Fiber: 4g
- Sugar: 6g

Number of Serves: 4
Cooking Time: 20 minutes

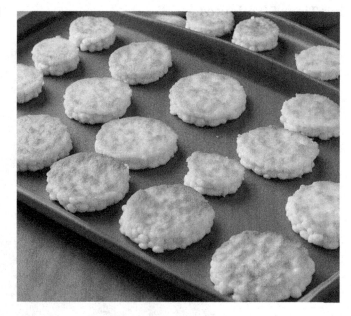

15. Steamed Vegetable Medley with Poached Eggs

Ingredients:

- 1 cup broccoli florets
- 1 cup cauliflower florets
- 1 cup baby carrots
- 4 large eggs
- 1 tablespoon olive oil
- 1 teaspoon dried thyme

Instructions:

1. Steam the broccoli, cauliflower, and baby carrots until tender, about 5-7 minutes. Set aside.
2. Fill a large saucepan with 2-3 inches of water and bring to a simmer over medium heat.
3. Crack each egg into a small bowl and gently slide them into the simmering water.
4. Poach the eggs for 3-4 minutes, or until the whites are set and the yolks are still runny.
5. Divide the steamed vegetables among four plates and drizzle with olive oil. Sprinkle with dried thyme.
6. Top each plate with a poached egg.
7. Serve warm.

Nutrition Info per Serving:

- Calories: 170
- Protein: 9g
- Carbohydrates: 10g
- Fat: 10g
- Fiber: 4g
- Sugar: 4g

Number of Serves: 4
Cooking Time: 15 minutes

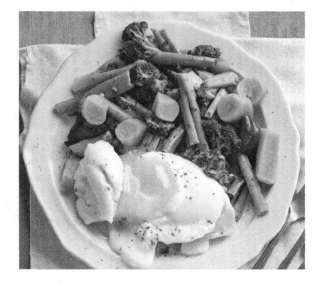

16. Quinoa Breakfast Bowl

Ingredients:

- 1 cup quinoa
- 2 cups water
- 1 cup almond milk (unsweetened)
- 1 tablespoon honey
- 1 teaspoon vanilla extract
- 1/2 cup fresh berries (blueberries, strawberries, or raspberries)
- 1/4 cup chopped nuts (almonds, walnuts, or pecans)
- 1 tablespoon chia seeds

Instructions:

1. Rinse the quinoa under cold water.
2. In a medium saucepan, combine the quinoa and water. Bring to a boil over medium heat.
3. Reduce the heat to low, cover, and simmer for 15 minutes, or until the quinoa is tender and the water is absorbed.
4. Stir in the almond milk, honey, and vanilla extract. Cook for an additional 5 minutes until heated through.
5. Divide the quinoa mixture into bowls and top with fresh berries, chopped nuts, and chia seeds.
6. Serve warm.

Nutrition Info per Serving:

- Calories: 300
- Protein: 8g
- Carbohydrates: 44g
- Fat: 10g
- Fiber: 6g
- Sugar: 10g

Number of Serves: 2
Cooking Time: 25 minutes

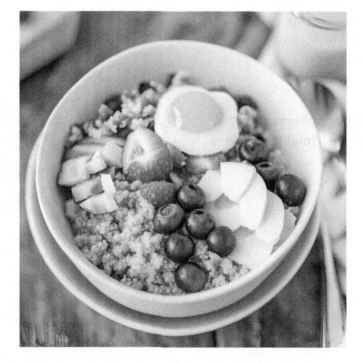

17. Chicken Congee

Ingredients:

- 1/2 cup jasmine rice
- 6 cups low-sodium chicken broth
- 1 cup cooked chicken breast, shredded
- 1 tablespoon fresh ginger, grated
- 2 green onions, chopped
- 1 tablespoon sesame oil
- 1 teaspoon low-sodium soy sauce

Instructions:

1. In a large pot, combine the jasmine rice, chicken broth, and grated ginger. Bring to a boil over medium-high heat.
2. Reduce the heat to low and simmer, stirring occasionally, for 1 to 1.5 hours, or until the rice has broken down and the congee has a porridge-like consistency.
3. Stir in the shredded chicken and cook for an additional 5 minutes.
4. Ladle the congee into bowls and top with chopped green onions, a drizzle of sesame oil, and soy sauce.
5. Serve warm.

Nutrition Info per Serving:

- Calories: 250
- Protein: 18g
- Carbohydrates: 32g
- Fat: 6g
- Fiber: 1g
- Sugar: 1g

Number of Serves: 4
Cooking Time: 1.5 hours

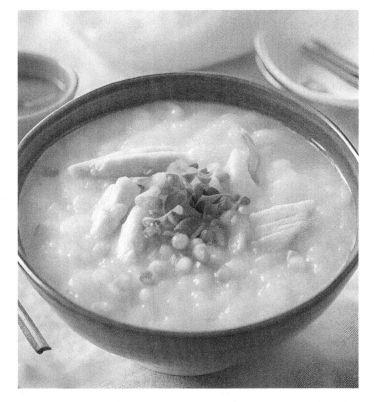

18. Peanut Butter Banana Smoothie

Ingredients:

- 1 banana, sliced and frozen
- 1 cup almond milk (unsweetened)
- 2 tablespoons natural peanut butter
- 1 tablespoon honey
- 1 teaspoon vanilla extract
- 1/4 teaspoon ground cinnamon

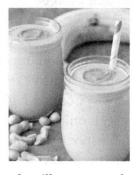

Instructions:

1. In a blender, combine the frozen banana slices, almond milk, peanut butter, honey, vanilla extract, and ground cinnamon.
2. Blend until smooth and creamy.
3. Pour into glasses and serve immediately.

Nutrition Info per Serving:

- Calories: 250 Protein: 6g Carbohydrates: 35g Fat: 10g Fiber: 4g Sugar: 18g

Number of Serves: 2

Cooking Time: 5 minutes

19. Greek Yogurt Parfait

Ingredients:

- 2 cups plain Greek yogurt
- 1/2 cup granola
- 1 cup mixed berries (blueberries, strawberries, raspberries)
- 2 tablespoons honey
- 1 teaspoon vanilla extract

Instructions:

1. In a bowl, mix the Greek yogurt, honey, and vanilla extract until well combined.
2. In serving glasses or bowls, layer the Greek yogurt mixture, granola, and mixed berries.
3. Repeat the layers until all ingredients are used.
4. Serve immediately.

Nutrition Info per Serving:

- Calories: 220
- Protein: 12g
- Carbohydrates: 34g
- Fat: 6g
- Fiber: 4g
- Sugar: 22g

Number of Serves: 2

Cooking Time: 10 minutes

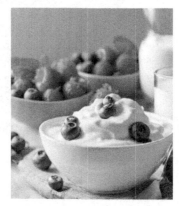

20. Sweet Potato Hash with Soft Cooked Eggs

Ingredients:

- 2 medium sweet potatoes, peeled and cubed
- 1 small onion, finely chopped
- 1 red bell pepper, chopped
- 1 tablespoon olive oil
- 4 large eggs
- 1 teaspoon dried thyme

Instructions:

1. In a large skillet, heat the olive oil over medium heat. Add the sweet potatoes, onion, and red bell pepper. Cook, stirring occasionally, until the sweet potatoes are tender and slightly crispy, about 15-20 minutes.
2. While the hash is cooking, bring a pot of water to a simmer. Carefully lower the eggs into the water and cook for 6 minutes for soft-cooked eggs.
3. Remove the eggs from the water and place them in a bowl of ice water to cool slightly. Peel the eggs.
4. Sprinkle the dried thyme over the sweet potato hash and stir to combine.
5. Divide the hash among four plates and top each serving with a soft-cooked egg.
6. Serve warm.

Nutrition Info per Serving:

- Calories: 250
- Protein: 9g
- Carbohydrates: 30g
- Fat: 12g
- Fiber: 5g
- Sugar: 7g

Number of Serves: 4

Cooking Time: 25 minutes

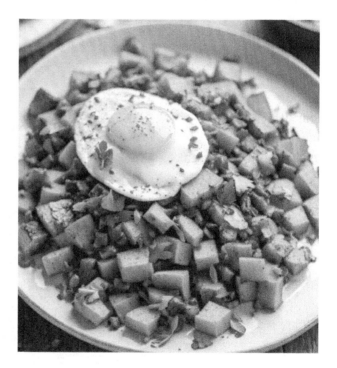

21. Pumpkin Porridge

Ingredients:

- 1 cup rolled oats
- 2 cups almond milk (unsweetened)
- 1 cup pumpkin puree
- 1 tablespoon honey
- 1 teaspoon ground cinnamon
- 1/2 teaspoon ground ginger
- 1/4 teaspoon ground nutmeg
- 1/4 cup chopped walnuts

Instructions:

1. In a medium saucepan, combine the rolled oats and almond milk. Bring to a boil over medium heat.
2. Reduce heat to low and stir in the pumpkin puree, honey, ground cinnamon, ground ginger, and ground nutmeg. Cook, stirring occasionally, until the oats are tender and the mixture is creamy, about 5-7 minutes.
3. Divide the porridge into bowls and top with chopped walnuts.
4. Serve warm.

Nutrition Info per Serving:

- Calories: 220
- Protein: 6g
- Carbohydrates: 35g
- Fat: 8g
- Fiber: 6g
- Sugar: 10g

Number of Serves: 4
Cooking Time: 10 minutes

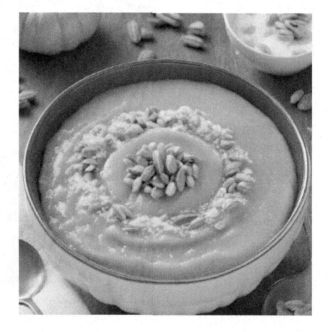

22. Mashed Potato Bowl with Scrambled Eggs

Ingredients:

- 4 medium potatoes, peeled and cubed
- 1/2 cup almond milk (unsweetened)
- 2 tablespoons olive oil
- 4 large eggs
- 1/4 cup plain Greek yogurt
- 1 tablespoon fresh chives, chopped

Instructions:

1. In a large pot, cover the potatoes with water and bring to a boil. Cook until tender, about 15 minutes.
2. Drain the potatoes and return them to the pot. Add the almond milk and 1 tablespoon of olive oil. Mash until smooth.
3. In a bowl, whisk the eggs.
4. Heat the remaining olive oil in a non-stick skillet over medium heat. Pour in the eggs and cook, stirring gently, until the eggs are scrambled and cooked through.
5. Divide the mashed potatoes among four bowls. Top each with a portion of scrambled eggs and a dollop of Greek yogurt.
6. Sprinkle with chopped chives and serve warm.

Nutrition Info per Serving:

- Calories: 250
- Protein: 10g
- Carbohydrates: 35g
- Fat: 10g
- Fiber: 5g
- Sugar: 4g

Number of Serves: 4

Cooking Time: 20 minutes

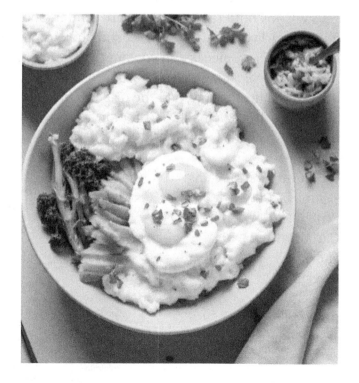

Poultry Recipes

1. Ginger Chicken Soup

Ingredients:

- 1 lb (450g) boneless, skinless chicken breasts, cut into small pieces
- 1 medium onion, finely chopped
- 2 carrots, sliced
- 2 celery stalks, sliced
- 2 cloves garlic, minced
- 1 tablespoon fresh ginger, grated
- 8 cups low-sodium chicken broth
- 1 tablespoon olive oil
- 1 teaspoon dried thyme
- 1 cup baby spinach
- Juice of 1 lemon

Instructions:

1. In a large pot, heat the olive oil over medium heat. Add the onion, carrots, and celery. Cook until the vegetables are tender, about 5 minutes.
2. Add the garlic and grated ginger, and cook for another 2 minutes.
3. Add the chicken pieces and cook until they are no longer pink on the outside.
4. Pour in the chicken broth and bring to a boil.
5. Reduce the heat to low, add the dried thyme, and simmer for 20 minutes.
6. Stir in the baby spinach and lemon juice. Cook for an additional 2-3 minutes until the spinach is wilted.
7. Serve hot.

Nutrition Info per Serving:

- Calories: 200
- Protein: 30g
- Carbohydrates: 10g
- Fat: 5g
- Fiber: 2g
- Sugar: 4g

Number of Serves: 4
Cooking Time: 30 minutes

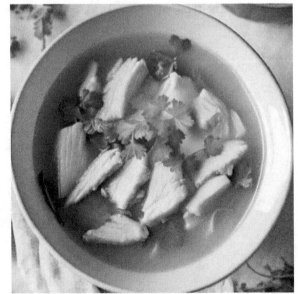

2. Turkey and Sweet Potato Stew

Ingredients:

- 1 lb (450g) turkey breast, cut into cubes
- 2 medium sweet potatoes, peeled and cubed
- 1 medium onion, chopped
- 2 cloves garlic, minced
- 1 red bell pepper, chopped
- 1 can (14.5 oz) diced tomatoes, no salt added
- 4 cups low-sodium chicken broth
- 1 tablespoon olive oil
- 1 teaspoon dried oregano
- 1 teaspoon ground cumin

Instructions:

1. In a large pot, heat the olive oil over medium heat. Add the onion and cook until softened, about 5 minutes.
2. Add the garlic and turkey cubes, cooking until the turkey is browned on all sides.
3. Stir in the sweet potatoes, red bell pepper, diced tomatoes, chicken broth, oregano, and cumin.
4. Bring the stew to a boil, then reduce the heat to low and simmer for 25-30 minutes, or until the sweet potatoes are tender.
5. Serve warm.

Nutrition Info per Serving:

- Calories: 250
- Protein: 25g
- Carbohydrates: 28g
- Fat: 5g
- Fiber: 6g
- Sugar: 10g

Number of Serves: 4
Cooking Time: 40 minutes

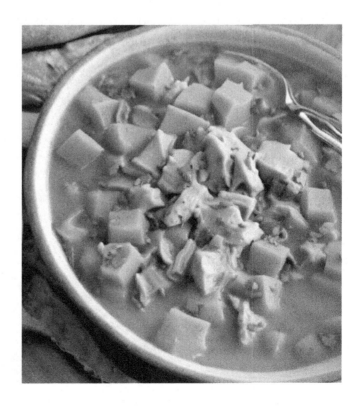

3. Creamy Turkey Casserole

Ingredients:

- 2 cups cooked turkey breast, shredded
- 2 cups broccoli florets
- 1 medium onion, chopped
- 2 cloves garlic, minced
- 1 cup cooked quinoa
- 1 cup plain Greek yogurt
- 1/2 cup low-sodium chicken broth
- 1/2 cup shredded cheddar cheese
- 1 tablespoon olive oil
- 1 teaspoon dried thyme

Instructions:

1. Preheat the oven to 350°F (175°C).
2. In a large skillet, heat the olive oil over medium heat. Add the onion and cook until softened, about 5 minutes.
3. Add the garlic and broccoli, cooking until the broccoli is tender, about 5 minutes.
4. In a large bowl, combine the shredded turkey, cooked quinoa, Greek yogurt, chicken broth, and dried thyme.
5. Stir in the cooked onion and broccoli.
6. Transfer the mixture to a baking dish and top with shredded cheddar cheese.
7. Bake for 25-30 minutes, or until the casserole is heated through and the cheese is melted.
8. Serve warm.

Nutrition Info per Serving:

- Calories: 300
- Protein: 30g
- Carbohydrates: 20g
- Fat: 10g
- Fiber: 4g
- Sugar: 4g

Number of Serves: 4

Cooking Time: 40 minutes

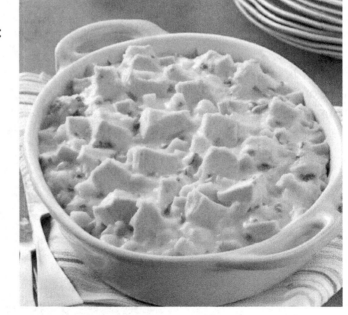

4. Turkey Meatballs in Tomato Sauce

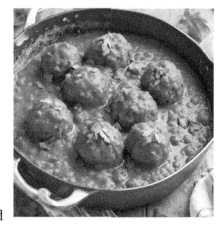

Ingredients:

- **For the Meatballs:**
  - 1 lb (450g) ground turkey
  - 1/2 cup whole wheat breadcrumbs
  - 1 large egg
  - 2 cloves garlic, minced
  - 1 tablespoon dried oregano
  - 1/4 cup grated Parmesan cheese
- For the Tomato Sauce:
  - 1 can (28 oz) crushed tomatoes, no salt added
  - 1 medium onion, finely chopped
  - 2 cloves garlic, minced
  - 1 tablespoon olive oil
  - 1 teaspoon dried basil

Instructions:

1. **To make the Meatballs:**
   - In a large bowl, combine the ground turkey, whole wheat breadcrumbs, egg, minced garlic, dried oregano, and grated Parmesan cheese. Mix until well combined.
   - Form the mixture into small meatballs, about 1 inch in diameter.
   - Place the meatballs on a baking sheet lined with parchment paper and bake at 375°F (190°C) for 15-20 minutes, or until fully cooked.
2. **To make the Tomato Sauce:**
   - In a large skillet, heat the olive oil over medium heat. Add the chopped onion and cook until softened, about 5 minutes.
   - Add the minced garlic and cook for another 2 minutes.
   - Stir in the crushed tomatoes and dried basil. Bring to a simmer and cook for 15-20 minutes, stirring occasionally.
3. **To combine:**
   - Add the baked meatballs to the tomato sauce and simmer for an additional 5 minutes to allow the flavors to meld.
   - Serve warm.

Nutrition Info per Serving:

- Calories: 280 Protein: 28g Carbohydrates: 20g
- Fat: 12g Fiber: 4g Sugar: 7g

Number of Serves: 4
Cooking Time: 40 minutes

5. Chicken Pot Pie with Biscuit Topping

Ingredients:

- **For the Filling:**
    - 1 lb (450g) boneless, skinless chicken breasts, cubed
    - 2 cups low-sodium chicken broth
    - 1 cup carrots, diced   1 cup peas (fresh or frozen)   1 cup celery, diced
    - 1 medium onion, chopped   2 cloves garlic, minced
    - 1 cup almond milk (unsweetened)
    - 1/4 cup whole wheat flour
    - 2 tablespoons olive oil
    - 1 teaspoon dried thyme
- **For the Biscuit Topping:**
    - 1 1/2 cups whole wheat flour
    - 1 tablespoon baking powder
    - 1/2 teaspoon baking soda
    - 1/2 cup almond milk (unsweetened)
    - 1/4 cup olive oil

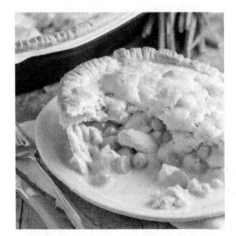

Instructions:

1. To make the Filling:
    - In a large pot, heat the olive oil over medium heat. Add the chicken cubes and cook until browned on all sides.
    - Remove the chicken and set aside. In the same pot, add the onion, garlic, carrots, celery, and peas. Cook until the vegetables are tender, about 5 minutes.
    - Sprinkle the whole wheat flour over the vegetables and stir well to coat. Gradually add the chicken broth and almond milk, stirring continuously until the mixture thickens.
    - Return the chicken to the pot and add the dried thyme. Simmer for 5-10 minutes, until the mixture is well combined and heated through.
2. To make the Biscuit Topping:
    - Preheat the oven to 400°F (200°C).
    - In a large bowl, combine the whole wheat flour, baking powder, and baking soda.
    - Add the almond milk and olive oil, stirring until just combined.
    - Drop spoonfuls of the biscuit dough onto the chicken mixture in the pot.
3. To assemble and bake:
    - Transfer the pot to the oven and bake for 20-25 minutes, or until the biscuit topping is golden brown.
    - Serve warm.

Nutrition Info per Serving:
Calories: 350 Protein: 25g Carbohydrates: 40g Fat: 12g Fiber: 6g Sugar: 4g
Number of Serves: 6
Cooking Time: 45 minutes

6. Lemon Turkey Breast

Ingredients:

- 1 lb (450g) turkey breast
- 2 lemons, juiced and zested
- 2 cloves garlic, minced
- 2 tablespoons olive oil
- 1 teaspoon dried rosemary

Instructions:

1. Preheat the oven to 375°F (190°C).
2. In a small bowl, mix the lemon juice, lemon zest, minced garlic, olive oil, and dried rosemary.
3. Place the turkey breast in a baking dish and pour the lemon mixture over it.
4. Bake for 30-35 minutes, or until the turkey is cooked through and the internal temperature reaches 165°F (75°C).
5. Let the turkey rest for a few minutes before slicing.
6. Serve warm.

Nutrition Info per Serving:

- Calories: 200
- Protein: 30g
- Carbohydrates: 4g
- Fat: 7g
- Fiber: 1g
- Sugar: 1g

Number of Serves: 4
Cooking Time: 35 minutes

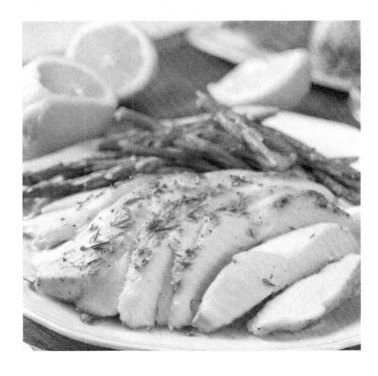

7. Chicken Noodle Soup

Ingredients:

- 1 lb (450g) boneless, skinless chicken breasts, cubed
- 8 cups low-sodium chicken broth
- 2 cups carrots, sliced
- 2 cups celery, sliced
- 1 medium onion, chopped
- 2 cloves garlic, minced
- 1 cup egg noodles
- 1 tablespoon olive oil
- 1 teaspoon dried thyme

Instructions:

1. In a large pot, heat the olive oil over medium heat. Add the onion, garlic, carrots, and celery. Cook until the vegetables are tender, about 5 minutes.
2. Add the cubed chicken and cook until browned on all sides.
3. Pour in the chicken broth and bring to a boil.
4. Add the egg noodles and dried thyme. Reduce the heat to low and simmer for 10-15 minutes, or until the noodles are tender and the chicken is cooked through.
5. Serve hot.

Nutrition Info per Serving:

- Calories: 250
- Protein: 25g
- Carbohydrates: 20g
- Fat: 8g
- Fiber: 3g
- Sugar: 4g

Number of Serves: 4
Cooking Time: 30 minutes

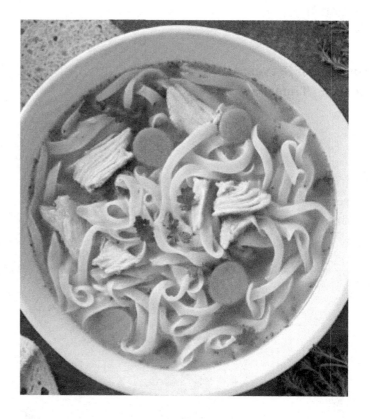

8. Chicken Porridge with Vegetables

Ingredients:

- 1 cup jasmine rice
- 6 cups low-sodium chicken broth
- 1 lb (450g) boneless, skinless chicken breasts, shredded
- 1 cup carrots, diced
- 1 cup celery, diced
- 1 tablespoon fresh ginger, grated
- 2 green onions, chopped
- 1 tablespoon olive oil

Instructions:

1. In a large pot, heat the olive oil over medium heat. Add the carrots, celery, and grated ginger. Cook until the vegetables are tender, about 5 minutes.
2. Add the jasmine rice and chicken broth. Bring to a boil.
3. Reduce the heat to low and simmer, stirring occasionally, for 1 to 1.5 hours, or until the rice has broken down and the porridge has a creamy consistency.
4. Stir in the shredded chicken and cook for an additional 5 minutes.
5. Garnish with chopped green onions and serve warm.

Nutrition Info per Serving:

- Calories: 300
- Protein: 25g
- Carbohydrates: 35g
- Fat: 8g
- Fiber: 3g
- Sugar: 2g

Number of Serves: 4
Cooking Time: 1.5 hours

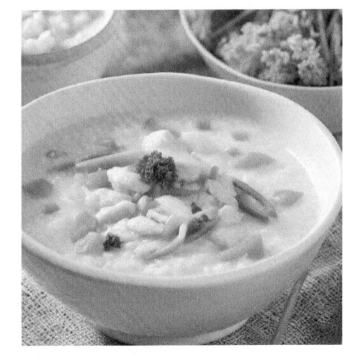

9. Baked Chicken with Apricot

Ingredients:

- 1 lb (450g) boneless, skinless chicken breasts
- 1 cup apricot preserves (no sugar added)
- 2 tablespoons Dijon mustard
- 1 tablespoon olive oil
- 1 teaspoon dried thyme

Instructions:

1. Preheat the oven to 375°F (190°C).
2. In a small bowl, mix the apricot preserves, Dijon mustard, olive oil, and dried thyme.
3. Place the chicken breasts in a baking dish and spread the apricot mixture over them.
4. Bake for 25-30 minutes, or until the chicken is cooked through and the internal temperature reaches 165°F (75°C).
5. Serve warm.

Nutrition Info per Serving:

- Calories: 250
- Protein: 30g
- Carbohydrates: 20g
- Fat: 6g
- Fiber: 1g
- Sugar: 18g

Number of Serves: 4
Cooking Time: 30 minutes

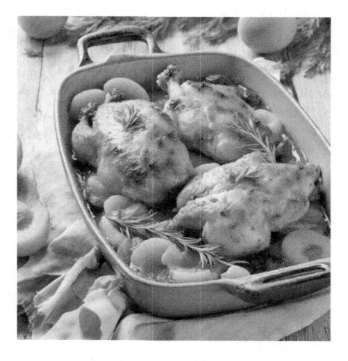

10. Turkey Sloppy Joes

Ingredients:

- 1 lb (450g) ground turkey
- 1 medium onion, chopped
- 1 green bell pepper, chopped
- 2 cloves garlic, minced
- 1 can (14.5 oz) tomato sauce, no salt added
- 2 tablespoons tomato paste
- 1 tablespoon Worcestershire sauce
- 1 teaspoon ground cumin
- 1 tablespoon olive oil
- 4 whole wheat buns

Instructions:

1. In a large skillet, heat the olive oil over medium heat. Add the chopped onion, green bell pepper, and garlic. Cook until the vegetables are tender, about 5 minutes.
2. Add the ground turkey and cook until browned.
3. Stir in the tomato sauce, tomato paste, Worcestershire sauce, and ground cumin. Bring to a simmer and cook for 10-15 minutes, or until the mixture thickens.
4. Serve the turkey mixture on whole wheat buns.

Nutrition Info per Serving:

- Calories: 350
- Protein: 25g
- Carbohydrates: 40g
- Fat: 10g
- Fiber: 6g
- Sugar: 10g

Number of Serves: 4
Cooking Time: 25 minutes

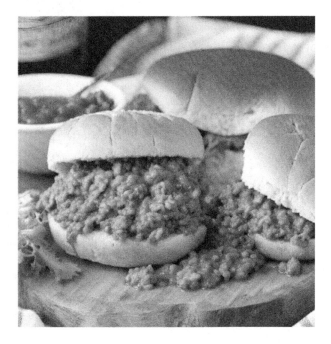

11. Turkey and Apple Burgers

Ingredients:

- 1 lb (450g) ground turkey
- 1 apple, peeled and grated
- 1 small onion, finely chopped
- 1/4 cup whole wheat breadcrumbs
- 1 large egg
- 1 teaspoon dried thyme
- 1 tablespoon olive oil
- 4 whole wheat buns

Instructions:

1. In a large bowl, combine the ground turkey, grated apple, chopped onion, whole wheat breadcrumbs, egg, and dried thyme. Mix until well combined.
2. Form the mixture into 4 patties.
3. In a large skillet, heat the olive oil over medium heat. Add the patties and cook for 5-7 minutes on each side, or until the burgers are cooked through and the internal temperature reaches 165°F (75°C).
4. Serve the burgers on whole wheat buns with desired toppings.

Nutrition Info per Serving:

- Calories: 300
- Protein: 28g
- Carbohydrates: 30g
- Fat: 10g
- Fiber: 4g
- Sugar: 6g

Number of Serves: 4
Cooking Time: 20 minutes

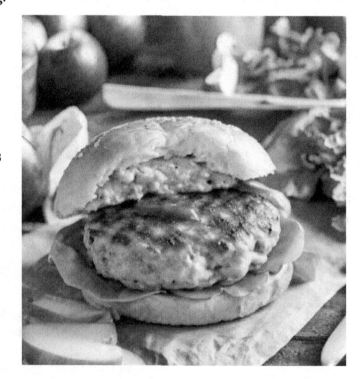

12. Poached Chicken Salad

Ingredients:

- 2 boneless, skinless chicken breasts
- 6 cups low-sodium chicken broth
- 1 cup cherry tomatoes, halved
- 1 cucumber, sliced
- 1 avocado, diced
- 4 cups mixed salad greens
- 2 tablespoons olive oil
- Juice of 1 lemon
- 1 teaspoon dried oregano

Instructions:

1. In a large pot, bring the chicken broth to a simmer. Add the chicken breasts and poach for 15-20 minutes, or until cooked through.
2. Remove the chicken from the broth and let cool. Shred the chicken into bite-sized pieces.
3. In a large bowl, combine the cherry tomatoes, cucumber, avocado, and mixed salad greens.
4. In a small bowl, whisk together the olive oil, lemon juice, and dried oregano.
5. Add the shredded chicken to the salad and drizzle with the dressing. Toss to combine.
6. Serve immediately.

Nutrition Info per Serving:

- Calories: 250
- Protein: 28g
- Carbohydrates: 10g
- Fat: 12g
- Fiber: 4g
- Sugar: 3g

Number of Serves: 4
Cooking Time: 25 minutes

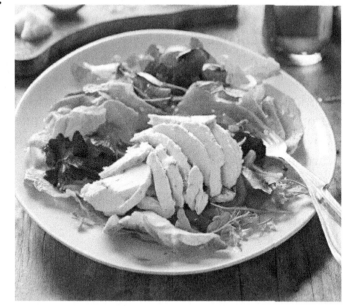

13. Chicken and Dumplings
Ingredients:
- **For the Chicken Soup:**
    - 1 lb (450g) boneless, skinless chicken breasts, cubed
    - 6 cups low-sodium chicken broth
    - 2 cups carrots, sliced
    - 2 cups celery, sliced
    - 1 medium onion, chopped
    - 2 cloves garlic, minced
    - 1 tablespoon olive oil
    - 1 teaspoon dried thyme
- For the Dumplings:
    - 1 cup whole wheat flour
    - 1 tablespoon baking powder
    - 1/2 teaspoon dried basil
    - 1/2 cup almond milk (unsweetened)
    - 2 tablespoons olive oil

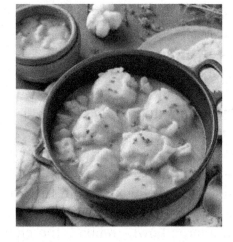

Instructions:
1. **To make the Chicken Soup:**
    - In a large pot, heat the olive oil over medium heat. Add the onion, garlic, carrots, and celery. Cook until the vegetables are tender, about 5 minutes.
    - Add the cubed chicken and cook until browned on all sides.
    - Pour in the chicken broth and bring to a boil. Reduce the heat to low, add the dried thyme, and simmer for 20 minutes.
2. **To make the Dumplings:**
    - In a medium bowl, combine the whole wheat flour, baking powder, and dried basil.
    - Stir in the almond milk and olive oil until just combined.
    - Drop spoonfuls of the dumpling batter into the simmering soup.
    - Cover the pot and cook for 15 minutes, or until the dumplings are cooked through.
3. To serve:
    - Ladle the soup and dumplings into bowls and serve hot.

Nutrition Info per Serving:
- Calories: 300
- Protein: 25g
- Carbohydrates: 30g
- Fat: 10g
- Fiber: 5g
- Sugar: 4g

Number of Serves: 4
Cooking Time: 40 minutes

14. Turkey and Spinach Quiche

Ingredients:

- 1 pre-made whole wheat pie crust
- 1 cup cooked turkey breast, shredded
- 2 cups fresh spinach, chopped
- 1/2 cup onion, finely chopped
- 1 cup almond milk (unsweetened)
- 4 large eggs
- 1/2 cup shredded mozzarella cheese
- 1 teaspoon dried thyme
- 1 tablespoon olive oil

Instructions:

1. Preheat the oven to 375°F (190°C).
2. In a skillet, heat the olive oil over medium heat. Add the chopped onion and cook until softened, about 5 minutes. Add the spinach and cook until wilted, about 2 minutes. Set aside to cool slightly.
3. In a large bowl, whisk together the eggs and almond milk. Stir in the shredded turkey, cooked spinach mixture, dried thyme, and shredded mozzarella cheese.
4. Pour the mixture into the pre-made whole wheat pie crust.
5. Bake for 35-40 minutes, or until the quiche is set and lightly golden on top.
6. Allow the quiche to cool slightly before slicing and serving.

Nutrition Info per Serving:

- Calories: 300
- Protein: 20g
- Carbohydrates: 22g
- Fat: 15g
- Fiber: 3g
- Sugar: 2g

Number of Serves: 6
Cooking Time: 45 minutes

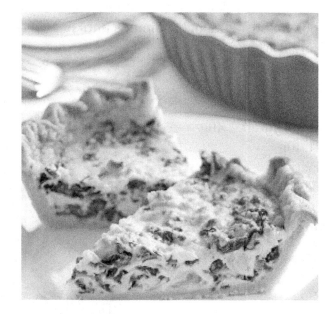

15. Chicken Risotto

Ingredients:

- 1 lb (450g) boneless, skinless chicken breasts, cubed
- 1 cup Arborio rice
- 1 small onion, finely chopped
- 2 cloves garlic, minced
- 4 cups low-sodium chicken broth
- 1/2 cup dry white wine (optional)
- 1/2 cup grated Parmesan cheese
- 1 cup peas (fresh or frozen)
- 1 tablespoon olive oil
- 1 teaspoon dried thyme

Instructions:

1. In a large pot, heat the olive oil over medium heat. Add the cubed chicken and cook until browned on all sides. Remove from the pot and set aside.
2. In the same pot, add the onion and garlic, and cook until softened, about 5 minutes.
3. Add the Arborio rice and cook for 1-2 minutes until slightly toasted.
4. Stir in the white wine (if using) and cook until absorbed.
5. Add the chicken broth one cup at a time, stirring frequently and allowing each addition to be absorbed before adding the next. Continue until the rice is creamy and tender, about 20 minutes.
6. Stir in the cooked chicken, peas, dried thyme, and grated Parmesan cheese. Cook for an additional 5 minutes until heated through.
7. Serve warm.

Nutrition Info per Serving:

- Calories: 350
- Protein: 28g
- Carbohydrates: 40g
- Fat: 10g
- Fiber: 3g
- Sugar: 2g

Number of Serves: 4
Cooking Time: 40 minutes

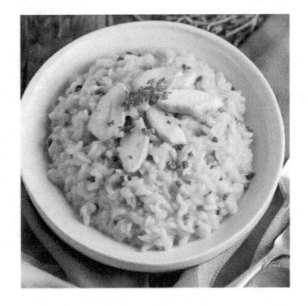

16. Slow Cooker Chicken Cacciatore

Ingredients:

- 1 lb (450g) boneless, skinless chicken thighs
- 1 large bell pepper, chopped
- 1 medium onion, chopped
- 2 cloves garlic, minced
- 1 can (28 oz) crushed tomatoes, no salt added
- 1/2 cup low-sodium chicken broth
- 1 tablespoon olive oil
- 1 teaspoon dried oregano
- 1 teaspoon dried basil
- 1 cup mushrooms, sliced

Instructions:

1. In a slow cooker, combine the chicken thighs, chopped bell pepper, onion, garlic, crushed tomatoes, chicken broth, olive oil, dried oregano, and dried basil.
2. Stir to combine, then cover and cook on low for 6-7 hours, or on high for 3-4 hours, until the chicken is tender.
3. About 30 minutes before serving, add the sliced mushrooms and continue to cook.
4. Serve warm, optionally over whole grain pasta or brown rice.

Nutrition Info per Serving:

- Calories: 250
- Protein: 28g
- Carbohydrates: 15g
- Fat: 10g
- Fiber: 4g
- Sugar: 7g

Number of Serves: 4
Cooking Time: 6-7 hours (slow cooker)

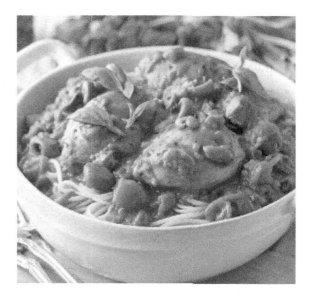

17. Turkey Shepherd's Pie

Ingredients:

- 1 lb (450g) ground turkey
- 2 cups mixed vegetables (carrots, peas, corn)
- 1 medium onion, chopped
- 2 cloves garlic, minced
- 2 cups mashed potatoes (prepared with almond milk and olive oil)
- 1 cup low-sodium chicken broth
- 1 tablespoon tomato paste
- 1 tablespoon olive oil
- 1 teaspoon dried thyme

Instructions:

1. Preheat the oven to 400°F (200°C).
2. In a large skillet, heat the olive oil over medium heat. Add the chopped onion and garlic, cooking until softened, about 5 minutes.
3. Add the ground turkey and cook until browned.
4. Stir in the mixed vegetables, chicken broth, tomato paste, and dried thyme. Simmer for 10 minutes, until the mixture thickens slightly.
5. Transfer the turkey mixture to a baking dish and spread evenly.
6. Spread the mashed potatoes over the top of the turkey mixture.
7. Bake for 20-25 minutes, until the top is lightly golden.
8. Serve warm.

Nutrition Info per Serving:

- Calories: 300
- Protein: 25g
- Carbohydrates: 30g
- Fat: 10g
- Fiber: 5g
- Sugar: 4g

Number of Serves: 4
Cooking Time: 35 minutes

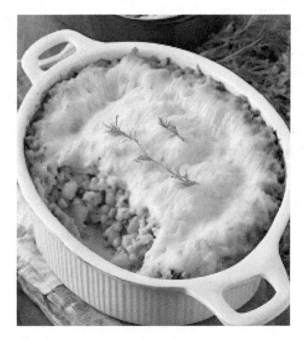

18. Balsamic Glazed Chicken

Ingredients:

- 1 lb (450g) boneless, skinless chicken breasts
- 1/4 cup balsamic vinegar
- 2 tablespoons honey
- 2 cloves garlic, minced
- 1 tablespoon olive oil
- 1 teaspoon dried rosemary

Instructions:

1. Preheat the oven to 400°F (200°C).
2. In a small bowl, mix the balsamic vinegar, honey, minced garlic, olive oil, and dried rosemary.
3. Place the chicken breasts in a baking dish and pour the balsamic mixture over them, ensuring they are well coated.
4. Bake for 25-30 minutes, or until the chicken is cooked through and the internal temperature reaches 165°F (75°C).
5. Let the chicken rest for a few minutes before serving. Spoon the balsamic glaze from the baking dish over the chicken.
6. Serve warm.

Nutrition Info per Serving:

- Calories: 210
- Protein: 28g
- Carbohydrates: 10g
- Fat: 7g
- Fiber: 0g
- Sugar: 8g

Number of Serves: 4
Cooking Time: 30 minutes

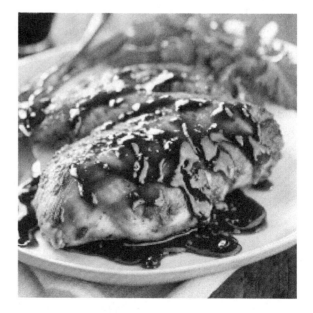

19. Turkey and Vegetable Loaf

Ingredients:

- 1 lb (450g) ground turkey
- 1 cup zucchini, grated
- 1 small onion, finely chopped
- 1 carrot, grated
- 2 cloves garlic, minced
- 1/2 cup whole wheat breadcrumbs
- 1 large egg
- 1/4 cup low-sodium chicken broth
- 1 tablespoon tomato paste
- 1 teaspoon dried thyme

Instructions:

1. Preheat the oven to 375°F (190°C).
2. In a large bowl, combine the ground turkey, grated zucchini, chopped onion, grated carrot, minced garlic, whole wheat breadcrumbs, egg, chicken broth, tomato paste, and dried thyme. Mix until well combined.
3. Transfer the mixture to a loaf pan and press down firmly to shape the loaf.
4. Bake for 45-50 minutes, or until the internal temperature reaches 165°F (75°C) and the loaf is cooked through.
5. Let the loaf rest for a few minutes before slicing and serving.
6. Serve warm.

Nutrition Info per Serving:

- Calories: 220
- Protein: 25g
- Carbohydrates: 10g
- Fat: 10g
- Fiber: 2g
- Sugar: 3g

Number of Serves: 4
Cooking Time: 50 minutes

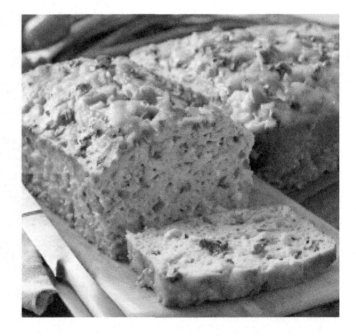

20. Creamy Chicken and Mushroom Pasta

Ingredients:

- 1 lb (450g) boneless, skinless chicken breasts, cubed
- 8 oz whole wheat pasta
- 2 cups mushrooms, sliced
- 1 small onion, finely chopped
- 2 cloves garlic, minced
- 1 cup almond milk (unsweetened)
- 1/2 cup low-sodium chicken broth
- 1/4 cup grated Parmesan cheese
- 1 tablespoon olive oil
- 1 teaspoon dried thyme

Instructions:

1. Cook the whole wheat pasta according to the package instructions. Drain and set aside.
2. In a large skillet, heat the olive oil over medium heat. Add the chopped onion and garlic, and cook until softened, about 5 minutes.
3. Add the cubed chicken and cook until browned on all sides.
4. Add the sliced mushrooms and cook until they are tender, about 5 minutes.
5. Pour in the almond milk and chicken broth, stirring to combine. Simmer for 10 minutes, until the sauce thickens slightly.
6. Stir in the grated Parmesan cheese and dried thyme.
7. Add the cooked pasta to the skillet and toss to combine with the sauce.
8. Serve warm.

Nutrition Info per Serving:

- Calories: 350
- Protein: 30g
- Carbohydrates: 40g
- Fat: 10g
- Fiber: 5g
- Sugar: 4g

Number of Serves: 4
Cooking Time: 30 minutes

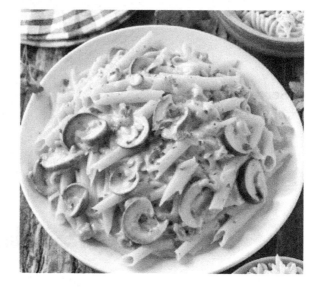

21. Turkey Piccata

Ingredients:

- 1 lb (450g) turkey breast cutlets
- 1/4 cup whole wheat flour
- 1/4 cup low-sodium chicken broth
- 1/4 cup lemon juice
- 2 tablespoons capers, rinsed and drained
- 2 tablespoons olive oil
- 1 tablespoon fresh parsley, chopped

Instructions:

1. Lightly coat the turkey breast cutlets with whole wheat flour, shaking off any excess.
2. In a large skillet, heat the olive oil over medium heat. Add the turkey cutlets and cook for 3-4 minutes on each side, until golden brown and cooked through.
3. Remove the turkey from the skillet and set aside.
4. In the same skillet, add the chicken broth, lemon juice, and capers. Bring to a simmer and cook for 2-3 minutes, until the sauce thickens slightly.
5. Return the turkey cutlets to the skillet and cook for an additional 2 minutes, until heated through and well coated with the sauce.
6. Sprinkle with fresh parsley before serving.
7. Serve warm.

Nutrition Info per Serving:

- Calories: 220
- Protein: 28g
- Carbohydrates: 8g
- Fat: 8g
- Fiber: 1g
- Sugar: 1g

Number of Serves: 4
Cooking Time: 20 minutes

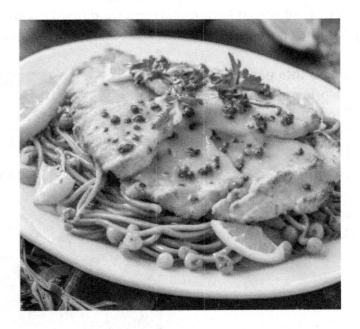

22. Orange Glazed Turkey

Ingredients:

- 1 lb (450g) turkey breast cutlets
- 1/2 cup orange juice (freshly squeezed)
- 1 tablespoon orange zest
- 2 tablespoons honey
- 2 cloves garlic, minced
- 1 tablespoon olive oil
- 1 teaspoon dried rosemary

Instructions:

1. In a small bowl, combine the orange juice, orange zest, honey, minced garlic, and dried rosemary.
2. In a large skillet, heat the olive oil over medium heat. Add the turkey breast cutlets and cook for 3-4 minutes on each side, until golden brown and cooked through.
3. Pour the orange juice mixture over the turkey cutlets and bring to a simmer. Cook for an additional 5 minutes, until the sauce thickens slightly and coats the turkey.
4. Serve warm.

Nutrition Info per Serving:

- Calories: 230
- Protein: 28g
- Carbohydrates: 12g
- Fat: 8g
- Fiber: 1g
- Sugar: 10g

Number of Serves: 4
Cooking Time: 15 minutes

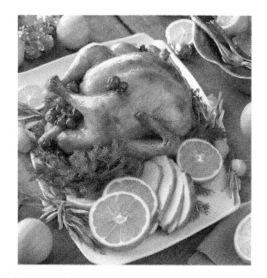

23. Smothered Turkey Wings

Ingredients:

- 2 lbs (900g) turkey wings, cut into sections
- 1 large onion, thinly sliced
- 2 cloves garlic, minced
- 2 cups low-sodium chicken broth
- 1 cup almond milk (unsweetened)
- 2 tablespoons whole wheat flour
- 2 tablespoons olive oil
- 1 teaspoon dried thyme

Instructions:

1. Preheat the oven to 350°F (175°C).
2. In a large skillet, heat the olive oil over medium heat. Add the turkey wings and cook until browned on all sides. Remove the turkey wings and set aside.
3. In the same skillet, add the sliced onion and minced garlic. Cook until the onions are softened, about 5 minutes.
4. Sprinkle the whole wheat flour over the onions and garlic, stirring well to coat. Gradually add the chicken broth and almond milk, stirring continuously until the mixture thickens.
5. Add the browned turkey wings back to the skillet, coating them with the sauce. Sprinkle with dried thyme.
6. Transfer the skillet to the oven and bake for 1.5 hours, or until the turkey wings are tender.
7. Serve warm.

Nutrition Info per Serving:

- Calories: 300
- Protein: 28g
- Carbohydrates: 10g
- Fat: 18g
- Fiber: 1g
- Sugar: 2g

Number of Serves: 4
Cooking Time: 1.5 hours

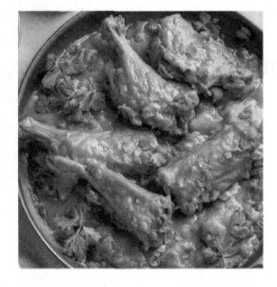

24. Chicken and Prune Tagine

Ingredients:

- 1 lb (450g) boneless, skinless chicken thighs
- 1 cup prunes, pitted and halved
- 1 medium onion, finely chopped
- 2 cloves garlic, minced
- 1 cup low-sodium chicken broth
- 1 tablespoon honey
- 1 teaspoon ground cinnamon
- 1 teaspoon ground cumin
- 1 tablespoon olive oil
- 1/4 cup sliced almonds

Instructions:

1. In a large pot or tagine, heat the olive oil over medium heat. Add the chopped onion and garlic, cooking until softened, about 5 minutes.
2. Add the chicken thighs and cook until browned on all sides.
3. Stir in the prunes, chicken broth, honey, ground cinnamon, and ground cumin.
4. Bring to a simmer, then cover and cook on low heat for 45 minutes, until the chicken is tender and the flavors are well combined.
5. Sprinkle with sliced almonds before serving.
6. Serve warm.

Nutrition Info per Serving:

- Calories: 320
- Protein: 28g
- Carbohydrates: 25g
- Fat: 12g
- Fiber: 4g
- Sugar: 18g

Number of Serves: 4
Cooking Time: 1 hour

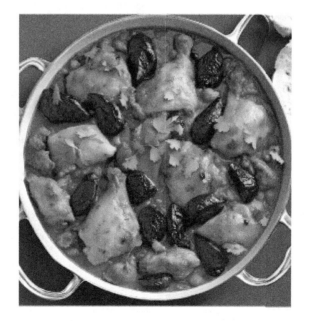

25. Turkey and Butternut Squash Hash

Ingredients:

- 1 lb (450g) ground turkey
- 2 cups butternut squash, peeled and cubed
- 1 small onion, finely chopped
- 1 red bell pepper, chopped
- 2 cloves garlic, minced
- 1 tablespoon olive oil
- 1 teaspoon dried sage

Instructions:

1. In a large skillet, heat the olive oil over medium heat. Add the ground turkey and cook until browned.
2. Add the chopped onion, red bell pepper, and garlic to the skillet, cooking until the vegetables are tender, about 5 minutes.
3. Stir in the butternut squash and dried sage. Cook for an additional 10-15 minutes, or until the squash is tender and lightly browned.
4. Serve warm.

Nutrition Info per Serving:

- Calories: 280
- Protein: 28g
- Carbohydrates: 20g
- Fat: 12g
- Fiber: 4g
- Sugar: 5g

Number of Serves: 4
Cooking Time: 25 minute

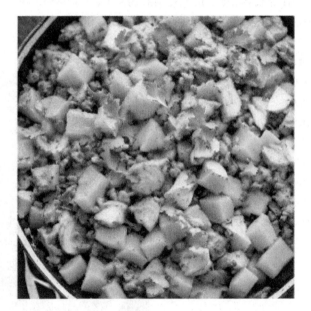

Fish & Seafood Recipes

1. Creamy Fish Chowder

Ingredients:

- 1 lb (450g) white fish fillets (such as cod or haddock), cut into chunks
- 1 cup almond milk (unsweetened)
- 2 cups low-sodium chicken broth
- 2 medium potatoes, peeled and diced
- 1 medium onion, finely chopped
- 2 cloves garlic, minced
- 1 cup corn kernels (fresh or frozen)
- 1 cup celery, diced
- 1 tablespoon olive oil
- 1 teaspoon dried thyme
- 1 bay leaf
- 1 tablespoon fresh parsley, chopped (optional)

Instructions:

1. In a large pot, heat the olive oil over medium heat. Add the onion and garlic, cooking until softened, about 5 minutes.
2. Add the potatoes, celery, and corn kernels, and cook for another 5 minutes.
3. Pour in the chicken broth and almond milk, and add the dried thyme and bay leaf. Bring to a boil.
4. Reduce the heat and simmer for 15-20 minutes, or until the potatoes are tender.
5. Add the fish chunks and cook for an additional 5-7 minutes, or until the fish is cooked through.
6. Remove the bay leaf and stir in the fresh parsley, if using.
7. Serve warm.

Nutrition Info per Serving:

- Calories: 250
- Protein: 25g
- Carbohydrates: 25g
- Fat: 8g
- Fiber: 3g
- Sugar: 5g

Number of Serves: 4
Cooking Time: 30 minutes

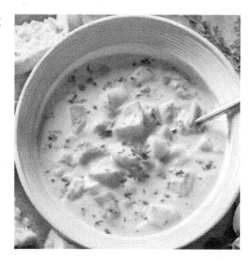

2. Lemon Tilapia with Herbed Quinoa

Ingredients:

- 4 tilapia fillets
- 2 lemons, juiced and zested
- 1 tablespoon olive oil
- 1 teaspoon dried oregano
- 1 cup quinoa
- 2 cups low-sodium chicken broth
- 1 cup cherry tomatoes, halved
- 1/4 cup fresh parsley, chopped
- 1/4 cup fresh basil, chopped

Instructions:

1. Preheat the oven to 375°F (190°C).
2. In a small bowl, mix the lemon juice, lemon zest, olive oil, and dried oregano.
3. Place the tilapia fillets in a baking dish and pour the lemon mixture over them. Bake for 15-20 minutes, or until the fish is cooked through.
4. While the fish is baking, rinse the quinoa under cold water. In a medium saucepan, bring the chicken broth to a boil. Add the quinoa, reduce the heat to low, and simmer for 15 minutes, or until the quinoa is tender and the liquid is absorbed.
5. Stir the cherry tomatoes, fresh parsley, and fresh basil into the cooked quinoa.
6. Serve the tilapia fillets over the herbed quinoa.

Nutrition Info per Serving:

- Calories: 350
- Protein: 30g
- Carbohydrates: 35g
- Fat: 10g
- Fiber: 5g
- Sugar: 4g

Number of Serves: 4
Cooking Time: 25 minutes

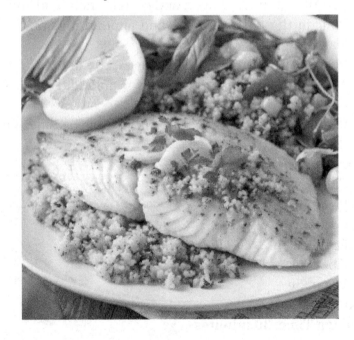

3. Shrimp and Rice Pilaf

Ingredients:

- 1 lb (450g) shrimp, peeled and deveined
- 1 cup basmati rice
- 2 cups low-sodium chicken broth
- 1 medium onion, finely chopped
- 2 cloves garlic, minced
- 1 cup peas (fresh or frozen)
- 1 red bell pepper, chopped
- 1 tablespoon olive oil
- 1 teaspoon dried thyme

Instructions:

1. In a large skillet, heat the olive oil over medium heat. Add the onion and garlic, cooking until softened, about 5 minutes.
2. Add the basmati rice and cook for 1-2 minutes until slightly toasted.
3. Pour in the chicken broth and bring to a boil. Reduce the heat, cover, and simmer for 15 minutes, or until the rice is tender and the liquid is absorbed.
4. In another skillet, cook the shrimp over medium heat until pink and opaque, about 3-4 minutes per side.
5. Stir the cooked shrimp, peas, and red bell pepper into the rice pilaf. Cook for an additional 5 minutes until the vegetables are tender.
6. Serve warm.

Nutrition Info per Serving:

- Calories: 300
- Protein: 25g
- Carbohydrates: 35g
- Fat: 8g
- Fiber: 4g
- Sugar: 3g

Number of Serves: 4
Cooking Time: 25 minutes

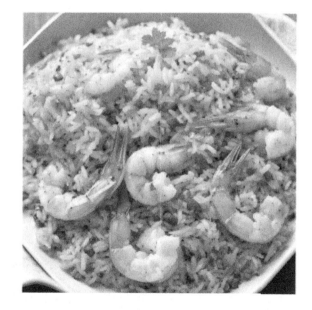

4. Cod in Papillote with Vegetables

Ingredients:

- 4 cod fillets
- 1 zucchini, thinly sliced
- 1 yellow squash, thinly sliced
- 1 red bell pepper, thinly sliced
- 1 medium onion, thinly sliced
- 2 cloves garlic, minced
- 2 lemons, thinly sliced
- 1 tablespoon olive oil
- 1 teaspoon dried thyme
- Parchment paper

Instructions:

1. Preheat the oven to 375°F (190°C).
2. Cut four large pieces of parchment paper.
3. In a small bowl, mix the olive oil, minced garlic, and dried thyme.
4. Place a cod fillet in the center of each piece of parchment paper. Arrange the zucchini, yellow squash, red bell pepper, and onion slices around the cod.
5. Drizzle the olive oil mixture over the cod and vegetables. Top each fillet with lemon slices.
6. Fold the parchment paper over the fish and vegetables to create a sealed packet.
7. Place the packets on a baking sheet and bake for 20-25 minutes, or until the fish is cooked through and the vegetables are tender.
8. Carefully open the packets and serve warm.

Nutrition Info per Serving:

- Calories: 250
- Protein: 30g
- Carbohydrates: 10g
- Fat: 10g
- Fiber: 3g
- Sugar: 4g

Number of Serves: 4
Cooking Time: 25 minutes

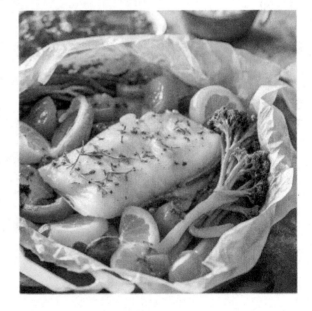

5. Seafood Pasta in White Sauce

Ingredients:

- 1 lb (450g) mixed seafood (shrimp, scallops, and calamari)
- 8 oz whole wheat pasta
- 1 cup almond milk (unsweetened)
- 1 cup low-sodium chicken broth
- 1/2 cup grated Parmesan cheese
- 1 tablespoon olive oil
- 2 cloves garlic, minced
- 1 small onion, finely chopped
- 1 tablespoon whole wheat flour
- 1 teaspoon dried basil

Instructions:

1. Cook the whole wheat pasta according to the package instructions. Drain and set aside.
2. In a large skillet, heat the olive oil over medium heat. Add the onion and garlic, and cook until softened, about 5 minutes.
3. Add the mixed seafood and cook until just opaque, about 3-4 minutes.
4. Sprinkle the whole wheat flour over the seafood and stir to coat. Gradually add the chicken broth and almond milk, stirring continuously until the sauce thickens.
5. Stir in the grated Parmesan cheese and dried basil. Simmer for 5 minutes.
6. Toss the cooked pasta with the seafood and sauce.
7. Serve warm.

Nutrition Info per Serving:

- Calories: 400
- Protein: 35g
- Carbohydrates: 40g
- Fat: 12g
- Fiber: 6g
- Sugar: 4g

Number of Serves: 4
Cooking Time: 30 minutes

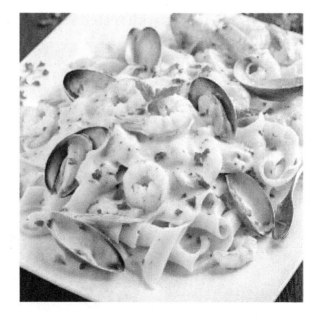

6. Pea and Mint Risotto with Scallops

Ingredients:

- 1 lb (450g) scallops
- 1 cup Arborio rice
- 4 cups low-sodium vegetable broth
- 1 cup peas (fresh or frozen)
- 1 small onion, finely chopped
- 2 cloves garlic, minced
- 1/2 cup dry white wine (optional)
- 1/4 cup grated Parmesan cheese
- 1 tablespoon olive oil
- 1/4 cup fresh mint leaves, chopped

Instructions:

1. In a large pot, heat the olive oil over medium heat. Add the onion and garlic, and cook until softened, about 5 minutes.
2. Add the Arborio rice and cook for 1-2 minutes until slightly toasted.
3. Pour in the white wine (if using) and cook until absorbed.
4. Gradually add the vegetable broth, one cup at a time, stirring frequently and allowing each addition to be absorbed before adding the next. Continue until the rice is creamy and tender, about 20 minutes.
5. Stir in the peas and grated Parmesan cheese. Cook for an additional 5 minutes until the peas are tender.
6. In a separate skillet, sear the scallops over medium-high heat for 2-3 minutes per side, until golden brown and cooked through.
7. Stir the fresh mint leaves into the risotto.
8. Serve the risotto topped with seared scallops.

Nutrition Info per Serving:

- Calories: 380
- Protein: 30g
- Carbohydrates: 45g
- Fat: 10g
- Fiber: 4g
- Sugar: 4g

Number of Serves: 4
Cooking Time: 30 minutes

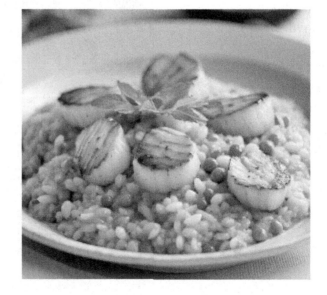

7. Salmon and Spinach Potato Casserole

Ingredients:

- 1 lb (450g) salmon fillets, skin removed and cubed
- 4 medium potatoes, peeled and thinly sliced
- 2 cups fresh spinach, chopped
- 1 small onion, finely chopped
- 1 cup almond milk (unsweetened)
- 1/2 cup low-sodium chicken broth
- 1/2 cup grated Parmesan cheese
- 1 tablespoon olive oil
- 1 teaspoon dried dill

Instructions:

1. Preheat the oven to 375°F (190°C).
2. In a large skillet, heat the olive oil over medium heat. Add the onion and cook until softened, about 5 minutes.
3. Layer the sliced potatoes in a greased baking dish. Top with the chopped spinach and cubed salmon.
4. In a small bowl, mix the almond milk, chicken broth, grated Parmesan cheese, and dried dill.
5. Pour the mixture over the layered potatoes, spinach, and salmon.
6. Cover the baking dish with foil and bake for 35-40 minutes, or until the potatoes are tender and the salmon is cooked through.
7. Remove the foil and bake for an additional 10 minutes, or until the top is lightly browned.
8. Serve warm.

Nutrition Info per Serving:

- Calories: 350
- Protein: 28g
- Carbohydrates: 35g
- Fat: 12g
- Fiber: 5g
- Sugar: 3g

Number of Serves: 4
Cooking Time: 50 minutes

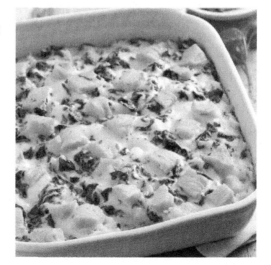

8. Poached Pear and Shrimp Salad

Ingredients:

- 1 lb (450g) shrimp, peeled and deveined
- 4 pears, peeled, cored, and halved
- 6 cups mixed salad greens
- 1/2 cup walnuts, chopped
- 1/4 cup crumbled feta cheese
- 1/2 cup pomegranate seeds (optional)
- 1 cup low-sodium vegetable broth
- 1 tablespoon honey
- 1 tablespoon lemon juice
- 1 tablespoon olive oil
- 1 teaspoon dried thyme

Instructions:

1. In a large pot, bring the vegetable broth, honey, and lemon juice to a simmer. Add the pear halves and poach for 15-20 minutes, or until tender. Remove the pears and let cool.
2. In a skillet, heat the olive oil over medium heat. Add the shrimp and dried thyme, cooking until the shrimp are pink and opaque, about 3-4 minutes per side.
3. Arrange the mixed salad greens on plates. Top with poached pear halves, cooked shrimp, chopped walnuts, crumbled feta cheese, and pomegranate seeds, if using.
4. Serve immediately.

Nutrition Info per Serving:

- Calories: 300
- Protein: 25g
- Carbohydrates: 30g
- Fat: 12g
- Fiber: 6g
- Sugar: 18g

Number of Serves: 4
Cooking Time: 25 minutes

9. Miso Glazed Cod

Ingredients:

- 4 cod fillets
- 1/4 cup white miso paste
- 2 tablespoons honey
- 2 tablespoons rice vinegar
- 1 tablespoon sesame oil
- 1 tablespoon fresh ginger, grated
- 1 clove garlic, minced

Instructions:

1. In a small bowl, whisk together the miso paste, honey, rice vinegar, sesame oil, grated ginger, and minced garlic.
2. Place the cod fillets in a shallow dish and pour the miso mixture over them, ensuring they are well coated. Marinate for at least 30 minutes.
3. Preheat the oven to 400°F (200°C).
4. Arrange the cod fillets on a baking sheet lined with parchment paper. Bake for 15-20 minutes, or until the fish is cooked through and flakes easily with a fork.
5. Serve warm.

Nutrition Info per Serving:

- Calories: 250
- Protein: 28g
- Carbohydrates: 15g
- Fat: 8g
- Fiber: 1g
- Sugar: 10g

Number of Serves: 4

Cooking Time: 20 minutes (plus marinating time)

10. Salmon Quiche with Dill

Ingredients:

- 1 pre-made whole wheat pie crust
- 1 cup cooked salmon, flaked
- 1 cup fresh spinach, chopped
- 1/2 cup onion, finely chopped
- 1 cup almond milk (unsweetened)
- 4 large eggs
- 1/2 cup shredded Swiss cheese
- 1 tablespoon fresh dill, chopped
- 1 tablespoon olive oil

Instructions:

1. Preheat the oven to 375°F (190°C).
2. In a skillet, heat the olive oil over medium heat. Add the onion and cook until softened, about 5 minutes. Add the spinach and cook until wilted, about 2 minutes. Set aside to cool slightly.
3. In a large bowl, whisk together the eggs and almond milk. Stir in the flaked salmon, cooked spinach mixture, fresh dill, and shredded Swiss cheese.
4. Pour the mixture into the pre-made whole wheat pie crust.
5. Bake for 35-40 minutes, or until the quiche is set and lightly golden on top.
6. Allow the quiche to cool slightly before slicing and serving.

Nutrition Info per Serving:

- Calories: 320
- Protein: 20g
- Carbohydrates: 22g
- Fat: 18g
- Fiber: 2g
- Sugar: 2g

Number of Serves: 6
Cooking Time: 45 minutes

11. Garlic Butter Scallops

Ingredients:

- 1 lb (450g) scallops
- 2 tablespoons unsalted butter
- 2 cloves garlic, minced
- 1 tablespoon fresh parsley, chopped
- 1 lemon, juiced

Instructions:

1. Pat the scallops dry with paper towels.
2. In a large skillet, melt the butter over medium-high heat. Add the minced garlic and cook for 1 minute until fragrant.
3. Add the scallops in a single layer and cook for 2-3 minutes per side, until golden brown and opaque.
4. Remove the scallops from the skillet and drizzle with lemon juice. Sprinkle with fresh parsley.
5. Serve immediately.

Nutrition Info per Serving:

- Calories: 200
- Protein: 28g
- Carbohydrates: 2g
- Fat: 9g
- Fiber: 0g
- Sugar: 0g

Number of Serves: 4
Cooking Time: 10 minutes

12. Tuna Salad Stuffed Avocado

Ingredients:

- 2 large avocados, halved and pitted
- 1 can (5 oz) tuna, packed in water, drained
- 1/4 cup plain Greek yogurt
- 1 tablespoon lemon juice
- 1 tablespoon fresh parsley, chopped
- 1 small celery stalk, finely chopped
- 1 small carrot, grated

Instructions:

1. In a bowl, combine the drained tuna, Greek yogurt, lemon juice, fresh parsley, chopped celery, and grated carrot. Mix until well combined.
2. Spoon the tuna salad into the avocado halves.
3. Serve immediately.

Nutrition Info per Serving:

- Calories: 250
- Protein: 15g
- Carbohydrates: 12g
- Fat: 18g
- Fiber: 8g
- Sugar: 2g

Number of Serves: 4

Cooking Time: 10 minutes

13. Shrimp Fried Rice

Ingredients:

- 1 lb (450g) shrimp, peeled and deveined
- 2 cups cooked brown rice (preferably cooled)
- 1 cup peas and carrots (fresh or frozen)
- 1 small onion, finely chopped
- 2 cloves garlic, minced
- 2 large eggs, beaten
- 3 tablespoons low-sodium soy sauce
- 1 tablespoon olive oil
- 1 teaspoon grated ginger

Instructions:

1. In a large skillet or wok, heat the olive oil over medium-high heat. Add the onion, garlic, and grated ginger, and cook until softened, about 5 minutes.
2. Add the shrimp and cook until pink and opaque, about 3-4 minutes.
3. Push the shrimp to one side of the skillet and pour the beaten eggs into the other side. Scramble the eggs until fully cooked, then mix them with the shrimp.
4. Add the cooked brown rice, peas, and carrots. Stir to combine and cook for another 5 minutes until the vegetables are tender and the rice is heated through.
5. Pour the soy sauce over the mixture and stir to coat evenly.
6. Serve warm.

Nutrition Info per Serving:

- Calories: 350
- Protein: 28g
- Carbohydrates: 40g
- Fat: 10g
- Fiber: 5g
- Sugar: 3g

Number of Serves: 4
Cooking Time: 20 minutes

14. Salmon Patties with Cucumber Yogurt Sauce

Ingredients:

- **For the Salmon Patties:**
    - 1 lb (450g) canned salmon, drained and flaked
    - 1/2 cup whole wheat breadcrumbs
    - 1 large egg, beaten
    - 1 small onion, finely chopped
    - 1 tablespoon fresh dill, chopped
    - 1 tablespoon lemon juice
    - 1 tablespoon olive oil
- For the Cucumber Yogurt Sauce:
    - 1/2 cup plain Greek yogurt
    - 1/2 cucumber, grated and squeezed to remove excess moisture
    - 1 tablespoon lemon juice
    - 1 tablespoon fresh dill, chopped

Instructions:

1. To make the Salmon Patties:
    - In a large bowl, combine the flaked salmon, whole wheat breadcrumbs, beaten egg, chopped onion, fresh dill, and lemon juice. Mix until well combined.
    - Form the mixture into 8 patties.
    - In a large skillet, heat the olive oil over medium heat. Cook the patties for 3-4 minutes per side, until golden brown and cooked through.
2. To make the Cucumber Yogurt Sauce:
    - In a small bowl, mix the Greek yogurt, grated cucumber, lemon juice, and fresh dill until well combined.
3. To serve:
    - Serve the salmon patties warm, topped with the cucumber yogurt sauce.

Nutrition Info per Serving:

- Calories: 300
- Protein: 25g
- Carbohydrates: 15g
- Fat: 15g
- Fiber: 2g
- Sugar: 3g

Number of Serves: 4

Cooking Time: 20 minutes

16. Fish Pie with Mashed Potato Topping

Ingredients:

- 1 lb (450g) white fish fillets (such as cod or haddock), cut into chunks
- 4 medium potatoes, peeled and cubed
- 1 cup almond milk (unsweetened)
- 1 cup low-sodium chicken broth
- 1 cup peas and carrots (fresh or frozen)
- 1 small onion, finely chopped
- 2 cloves garlic, minced
- 1 tablespoon whole wheat flour
- 2 tablespoons olive oil
- 1 teaspoon dried thyme
- 1 tablespoon fresh parsley, chopped (optional)

Instructions:

1. Preheat the oven to 375°F (190°C).
2. In a large pot, boil the potatoes until tender, about 15 minutes. Drain and mash with half of the almond milk. Set aside.
3. In a skillet, heat the olive oil over medium heat. Add the onion and garlic, cooking until softened, about 5 minutes.
4. Stir in the whole wheat flour and cook for 1 minute. Gradually add the chicken broth and remaining almond milk, stirring until the mixture thickens.
5. Add the fish chunks, peas, carrots, and dried thyme. Cook for an additional 5 minutes.
6. Transfer the fish mixture to a baking dish. Spread the mashed potatoes evenly over the top.
7. Bake for 20-25 minutes, or until the top is lightly golden.
8. Garnish with fresh parsley, if using. Serve warm.

Nutrition Info per Serving:

- Calories: 320
- Protein: 25g
- Carbohydrates: 40g
- Fat: 8g
- Fiber: 6g
- Sugar: 4g

Number of Serves: 4

Cooking Time: 45 minutes

17. Grilled Trout with Herbs

Ingredients:

- 4 trout fillets
- 2 tablespoons olive oil
- 1 lemon, juiced and zested
- 1 tablespoon fresh dill, chopped
- 1 tablespoon fresh parsley, chopped
- 1 teaspoon dried thyme

Instructions:

1. Preheat the grill to medium-high heat.
2. In a small bowl, mix the olive oil, lemon juice, lemon zest, fresh dill, fresh parsley, and dried thyme.
3. Brush the trout fillets with the herb mixture.
4. Grill the trout fillets for 4-5 minutes per side, or until the fish is cooked through and flakes easily with a fork.
5. Serve warm.

Nutrition Info per Serving:

- Calories: 220
- Protein: 28g
- Carbohydrates: 2g
- Fat: 10g
- Fiber: 1g
- Sugar: 1g

Number of Serves: 4
Cooking Time: 10 minutes

18. Shrimp Risotto

Ingredients:

- 1 lb (450g) shrimp, peeled and deveined
- 1 cup Arborio rice
- 4 cups low-sodium chicken broth
- 1 small onion, finely chopped
- 2 cloves garlic, minced
- 1/2 cup dry white wine (optional)
- 1/2 cup grated Parmesan cheese
- 1 tablespoon olive oil
- 1 tablespoon fresh parsley, chopped

Instructions:

1. In a large pot, heat the olive oil over medium heat. Add the onion and garlic, cooking until softened, about 5 minutes.
2. Add the Arborio rice and cook for 1-2 minutes until slightly toasted.
3. Pour in the white wine (if using) and cook until absorbed.
4. Gradually add the chicken broth, one cup at a time, stirring frequently and allowing each addition to be absorbed before adding the next. Continue until the rice is creamy and tender, about 20 minutes.
5. Stir in the shrimp and cook until they are pink and opaque, about 5 minutes.
6. Stir in the grated Parmesan cheese and fresh parsley.
7. Serve warm.

Nutrition Info per Serving:

- Calories: 350
- Protein: 28g
- Carbohydrates: 45g
- Fat: 10g
- Fiber: 3g
- Sugar: 2g

Number of Serves: 4
Cooking Time: 30 minutes

19. Pan-Seared Tuna with Olive Tapenade

Ingredients:

- 4 tuna steaks
- 1 cup mixed olives, pitted and chopped
- 2 cloves garlic, minced
- 1 tablespoon capers, rinsed and drained
- 2 tablespoons olive oil
- 1 tablespoon lemon juice
- 1 teaspoon dried oregano

Instructions:

1. In a small bowl, mix the chopped olives, minced garlic, capers, olive oil, lemon juice, and dried oregano to make the tapenade.
2. In a large skillet, heat a small amount of olive oil over medium-high heat. Add the tuna steaks and sear for 2-3 minutes per side, until the outside is browned but the inside is still pink (cook longer if desired).
3. Serve the tuna steaks topped with the olive tapenade.
4. Serve warm.

Nutrition Info per Serving:

- Calories: 300
- Protein: 35g
- Carbohydrates: 4g
- Fat: 16g
- Fiber: 2g
- Sugar: 0g

Number of Serves: 4
Cooking Time: 10 minutes

20. Baked Snapper with Tomato and Basil

Ingredients:

- 4 snapper fillets
- 2 cups cherry tomatoes, halved
- 1/4 cup fresh basil, chopped
- 2 cloves garlic, minced
- 1 tablespoon olive oil
- 1 lemon, juiced

Instructions:

1. Preheat the oven to 375°F (190°C).
2. In a baking dish, place the snapper fillets. Arrange the cherry tomatoes and minced garlic around the fish.
3. Drizzle with olive oil and lemon juice. Sprinkle with fresh basil.
4. Bake for 20-25 minutes, or until the fish is cooked through and flakes easily with a fork.
5. Serve warm.

Nutrition Info per Serving:

- Calories: 250
- Protein: 30g
- Carbohydrates: 8g
- Fat: 12g
- Fiber: 2g
- Sugar: 4g

Number of Serves: 4
Cooking Time: 25 minutes

21. Pasta with Clams and Light Garlic Sauce

Ingredients:

- 1 lb (450g) clams, cleaned
- 8 oz whole wheat pasta
- 4 cloves garlic, minced
- 1 cup low-sodium chicken broth
- 1/4 cup white wine (optional)
- 2 tablespoons olive oil
- 1/4 cup fresh parsley, chopped
- 1 lemon, juiced

Instructions:

1. Cook the whole wheat pasta according to the package instructions. Drain and set aside.
2. In a large skillet, heat the olive oil over medium heat. Add the garlic and cook for 1 minute until fragrant.
3. Add the clams, chicken broth, and white wine (if using). Cover and cook for 5-7 minutes, or until the clams open.
4. Remove the clams with a slotted spoon and set aside. Discard any clams that do not open.
5. Add the cooked pasta to the skillet and toss with the sauce.
6. Return the clams to the skillet, drizzle with lemon juice, and sprinkle with fresh parsley.
7. Serve warm.

Nutrition Info per Serving:

- Calories: 350
- Protein: 20g
- Carbohydrates: 45g
- Fat: 10g
- Fiber: 6g
- Sugar: 2g

Number of Serves: 4
Cooking Time: 20 minutes

Soup & Stew Recipes

1. Creamy Butternut Squash Soup

Ingredients:

- 1 medium butternut squash, peeled, seeded, and cubed
- 1 medium onion, chopped
- 2 cloves garlic, minced
- 4 cups low-sodium vegetable broth
- 1 cup almond milk (unsweetened)
- 1 tablespoon olive oil
- 1 teaspoon ground nutmeg
- 1 teaspoon dried thyme

Instructions:

1. In a large pot, heat the olive oil over medium heat. Add the onion and garlic, and cook until softened, about 5 minutes.
2. Add the cubed butternut squash, vegetable broth, nutmeg, and thyme. Bring to a boil, then reduce the heat and simmer for 20-25 minutes, or until the squash is tender.
3. Use an immersion blender to puree the soup until smooth, or transfer to a blender in batches and blend until smooth.
4. Stir in the almond milk and heat through, but do not boil.
5. Serve warm.

Nutrition Info per Serving:

- Calories: 150
- Protein: 3g
- Carbohydrates: 28g
- Fat: 4g
- Fiber: 5g
- Sugar: 8g

Number of Serves: 4
Cooking Time: 30 Minutes

2. Barley and Mushroom Stew

Ingredients:

- 1 cup pearl barley
- 8 oz mushrooms, sliced
- 1 medium onion, chopped
- 2 cloves garlic, minced
- 4 cups low-sodium vegetable broth
- 2 cups water
- 2 carrots, sliced
- 2 celery stalks, sliced
- 1 tablespoon olive oil
- 1 teaspoon dried thyme
- 1 bay leaf

Instructions:

1. In a large pot, heat the olive oil over medium heat. Add the onion and garlic, cooking until softened, about 5 minutes.
2. Add the sliced mushrooms and cook until they release their juices and begin to brown, about 5 minutes.
3. Stir in the carrots and celery, cooking for another 3 minutes.
4. Add the barley, vegetable broth, water, thyme, and bay leaf. Bring to a boil, then reduce the heat and simmer for 45 minutes to 1 hour, or until the barley is tender.
5. Remove the bay leaf before serving.
6. Serve warm.

Nutrition Info per Serving:

- Calories: 200
- Protein: 5g
- Carbohydrates: 40g
- Fat: 4g
- Fiber: 8g
- Sugar: 6g

Number of Serves: 4
Cooking Time: 1 hour

3. Carrot and Ginger Puree Soup

Ingredients:

- 1 lb (450g) carrots, peeled and sliced
- 1 medium onion, chopped
- 2 cloves garlic, minced
- 1 tablespoon fresh ginger, grated
- 4 cups low-sodium vegetable broth
- 1 cup almond milk (unsweetened)
- 1 tablespoon olive oil
- 1 teaspoon ground cumin

Instructions:

1. In a large pot, heat the olive oil over medium heat. Add the onion, garlic, and grated ginger, cooking until softened, about 5 minutes.
2. Add the sliced carrots and cumin, cooking for another 3 minutes.
3. Pour in the vegetable broth and bring to a boil. Reduce the heat and simmer for 20-25 minutes, or until the carrots are tender.
4. Use an immersion blender to puree the soup until smooth, or transfer to a blender in batches and blend until smooth.
5. Stir in the almond milk and heat through, but do not boil.
6. Serve warm.

Nutrition Info per Serving:

- Calories: 140
- Protein: 3g
- Carbohydrates: 25g
- Fat: 4g
- Fiber: 5g
- Sugar: 10g

Number of Serves: 4
Cooking Time: 30 minutes

4. Lentil Soup with Spinach

Ingredients:

- 1 cup green or brown lentils, rinsed
- 1 medium onion, chopped
- 2 cloves garlic, minced
- 2 carrots, diced
- 2 celery stalks, diced
- 4 cups low-sodium vegetable broth
- 2 cups water
- 2 cups fresh spinach, chopped
- 1 tablespoon olive oil
- 1 teaspoon ground cumin
- 1 teaspoon dried thyme

Instructions:

1. In a large pot, heat the olive oil over medium heat. Add the onion and garlic, cooking until softened, about 5 minutes.
2. Add the carrots and celery, cooking for another 3 minutes.
3. Stir in the lentils, vegetable broth, water, cumin, and thyme. Bring to a boil, then reduce the heat and simmer for 30-35 minutes, or until the lentils are tender.
4. Stir in the chopped spinach and cook for another 5 minutes, until the spinach is wilted.
5. Serve warm.

Nutrition Info per Serving:

- Calories: 220
- Protein: 12g
- Carbohydrates: 35g
- Fat: 5g
- Fiber: 12g
- Sugar: 5g

Number of Serves: 4
Cooking Time: 45 minutes

5. Sweet Potato and Coconut Milk Soup

Ingredients:

- 2 large sweet potatoes, peeled and cubed
- 1 medium onion, chopped
- 2 cloves garlic, minced
- 4 cups low-sodium vegetable broth
- 1 can (14 oz) coconut milk
- 1 tablespoon olive oil
- 1 teaspoon ground ginger
- 1 teaspoon ground cinnamon

Instructions:

1. In a large pot, heat the olive oil over medium heat. Add the onion and garlic, cooking until softened, about 5 minutes.
2. Add the cubed sweet potatoes, vegetable broth, ground ginger, and ground cinnamon. Bring to a boil.
3. Reduce the heat and simmer for 20-25 minutes, or until the sweet potatoes are tender.
4. Use an immersion blender to puree the soup until smooth, or transfer to a blender in batches and blend until smooth.
5. Stir in the coconut milk and heat through.
6. Serve warm.

Nutrition Info per Serving:

- Calories: 250
- Protein: 3g
- Carbohydrates: 35g
- Fat: 12g
- Fiber: 6g
- Sugar: 9g

Number of Serves: 4
Cooking Time: 30 minutes

6. Tomato Basil Soup

Ingredients:

- 2 lbs (900g) tomatoes, chopped
- 1 medium onion, chopped
- 2 cloves garlic, minced
- 4 cups low-sodium vegetable broth
- 1 cup almond milk (unsweetened)
- 1 tablespoon olive oil
- 1/4 cup fresh basil, chopped
- 1 teaspoon dried oregano

Instructions:

1. In a large pot, heat the olive oil over medium heat. Add the onion and garlic, cooking until softened, about 5 minutes.
2. Add the chopped tomatoes, vegetable broth, and dried oregano. Bring to a boil.
3. Reduce the heat and simmer for 20-25 minutes, or until the tomatoes are tender.
4. Use an immersion blender to puree the soup until smooth, or transfer to a blender in batches and blend until smooth.
5. Stir in the almond milk and fresh basil, and heat through.
6. Serve warm.

Nutrition Info per Serving:

- Calories: 160
- Protein: 4g
- Carbohydrates: 20g
- Fat: 8g
- Fiber: 5g
- Sugar: 10g

Number of Serves: 4
Cooking Time: 30 minutes

7. Pumpkin and Apple Soup

Ingredients:

- 1 medium pumpkin, peeled, seeded, and cubed
- 2 apples, peeled, cored, and chopped
- 1 medium onion, chopped
- 2 cloves garlic, minced
- 4 cups low-sodium vegetable broth
- 1 cup almond milk (unsweetened)
- 1 tablespoon olive oil
- 1 teaspoon ground cinnamon
- 1/2 teaspoon ground nutmeg

Instructions:

1. In a large pot, heat the olive oil over medium heat. Add the onion and garlic, cooking until softened, about 5 minutes.
2. Add the cubed pumpkin, chopped apples, vegetable broth, ground cinnamon, and ground nutmeg. Bring to a boil.
3. Reduce the heat and simmer for 20-25 minutes, or until the pumpkin and apples are tender.
4. Use an immersion blender to puree the soup until smooth, or transfer to a blender in batches and blend until smooth.
5. Stir in the almond milk and heat through.
6. Serve warm.

Nutrition Info per Serving:

- Calories: 200
- Protein: 3g
- Carbohydrates: 35g
- Fat: 7g
- Fiber: 7g
- Sugar: 18g

Number of Serves: 4
Cooking Time: 30 minutes

8. Cauliflower and Turmeric Soup

Ingredients:

- 1 large head of cauliflower, chopped
- 1 medium onion, chopped
- 2 cloves garlic, minced
- 4 cups low-sodium vegetable broth
- 1 cup almond milk (unsweetened)
- 1 tablespoon olive oil
- 1 teaspoon ground turmeric
- 1/2 teaspoon ground cumin

Instructions:

1. In a large pot, heat the olive oil over medium heat. Add the onion and garlic, cooking until softened, about 5 minutes.
2. Add the chopped cauliflower, vegetable broth, ground turmeric, and ground cumin. Bring to a boil.
3. Reduce the heat and simmer for 20-25 minutes, or until the cauliflower is tender.
4. Use an immersion blender to puree the soup until smooth, or transfer to a blender in batches and blend until smooth.
5. Stir in the almond milk and heat through.
6. Serve warm.

Nutrition Info per Serving:

- Calories: 180
- Protein: 4g
- Carbohydrates: 18g
- Fat: 10g
- Fiber: 6g
- Sugar: 6g

Number of Serves: 4
Cooking Time: 30 minutes

9. Potato Leek Soup

Ingredients:

- 4 medium potatoes, peeled and cubed
- 2 large leeks, cleaned and sliced
- 1 medium onion, chopped
- 2 cloves garlic, minced
- 4 cups low-sodium vegetable broth
- 1 cup almond milk (unsweetened)
- 1 tablespoon olive oil
- 1 teaspoon dried thyme

Instructions:

1. In a large pot, heat the olive oil over medium heat. Add the onion, garlic, and leeks, cooking until softened, about 5 minutes.
2. Add the cubed potatoes, vegetable broth, and dried thyme. Bring to a boil.
3. Reduce the heat and simmer for 20-25 minutes, or until the potatoes are tender.
4. Use an immersion blender to puree the soup until smooth, or transfer to a blender in batches and blend until smooth.
5. Stir in the almond milk and heat through.
6. Serve warm.

Nutrition Info per Serving:

- Calories: 220
- Protein: 4g
- Carbohydrates: 38g
- Fat: 7g
- Fiber: 6g
- Sugar: 5g

Number of Serves: 4

Cooking Time: 30 minutes

10. Cream of Asparagus Soup

Ingredients:

- 2 lbs (900g) asparagus, trimmed and chopped
- 1 medium onion, chopped
- 2 cloves garlic, minced
- 4 cups low-sodium vegetable broth
- 1 cup almond milk (unsweetened)
- 1 tablespoon olive oil
- 1 teaspoon dried tarragon

Instructions:

1. In a large pot, heat the olive oil over medium heat. Add the onion and garlic, cooking until softened, about 5 minutes.
2. Add the chopped asparagus, vegetable broth, and dried tarragon. Bring to a boil.
3. Reduce the heat and simmer for 15-20 minutes, or until the asparagus is tender.
4. Use an immersion blender to puree the soup until smooth, or transfer to a blender in batches and blend until smooth.
5. Stir in the almond milk and heat through.
6. Serve warm.

Nutrition Info per Serving:

- Calories: 180
- Protein: 5g
- Carbohydrates: 18g
- Fat: 9g
- Fiber: 5g
- Sugar: 5g

Number of Serves: 4
Cooking Time: 25 minutes

11. Miso Soup with Tofu

Ingredients:

- 4 cups water
- 1/4 cup miso paste
- 1 cup tofu, cubed
- 1 cup wakame seaweed, rehydrated
- 1 cup green onions, chopped
- 1 tablespoon soy sauce (low sodium)
- 1 teaspoon grated ginger

Instructions:

1. In a medium pot, bring the water to a boil.
2. Reduce the heat to low and whisk in the miso paste until fully dissolved.
3. Add the cubed tofu, wakame seaweed, soy sauce, and grated ginger.
4. Simmer for 5-7 minutes until the ingredients are heated through.
5. Stir in the chopped green onions just before serving.
6. Serve warm.

Nutrition Info per Serving:

- Calories: 80
- Protein: 5g
- Carbohydrates: 8g
- Fat: 3g
- Fiber: 1g
- Sugar: 2g

Number of Serves: 4
Cooking Time: 10 minutes

12. Borscht (Beet Soup)

Ingredients:

- 4 medium beets, peeled and grated
- 2 medium potatoes, peeled and cubed
- 1 medium carrot, peeled and grated
- 1 medium onion, chopped
- 2 cloves garlic, minced
- 6 cups low-sodium vegetable broth
- 1 cup cabbage, shredded
- 1 tablespoon tomato paste
- 1 tablespoon olive oil
- 1 teaspoon dried dill
- 1 tablespoon apple cider vinegar

Instructions:

1. In a large pot, heat the olive oil over medium heat. Add the onion and garlic, cooking until softened, about 5 minutes.
2. Add the grated beets, grated carrot, and cubed potatoes. Cook for another 5 minutes.
3. Stir in the tomato paste and cook for 1 minute.
4. Add the vegetable broth, shredded cabbage, and dried dill. Bring to a boil, then reduce the heat and simmer for 30 minutes.
5. Stir in the apple cider vinegar and cook for an additional 5 minutes.
6. Serve warm.

Nutrition Info per Serving:

- Calories: 150
- Protein: 4g
- Carbohydrates: 30g
- Fat: 3g
- Fiber: 6g
- Sugar: 10g

Number of Serves: 4
Cooking Time: 40 minutes

13. Split Pea Soup with Ham

Ingredients:

- 1 cup dried split peas, rinsed
- 1 cup ham, diced
- 1 medium onion, chopped
- 2 carrots, sliced
- 2 celery stalks, sliced
- 2 cloves garlic, minced
- 4 cups low-sodium chicken broth
- 2 cups water
- 1 tablespoon olive oil
- 1 teaspoon dried thyme

Instructions:

1. In a large pot, heat the olive oil over medium heat. Add the onion, garlic, carrots, and celery, cooking until softened, about 5 minutes.
2. Add the diced ham and cook for another 3 minutes.
3. Stir in the split peas, chicken broth, water, and dried thyme. Bring to a boil, then reduce the heat and simmer for 1 hour, or until the peas are tender.
4. Serve warm.

Nutrition Info per Serving:

- Calories: 250
- Protein: 18g
- Carbohydrates: 35g
- Fat: 6g
- Fiber: 12g
- Sugar: 5g

Number of Serves: 4
Cooking Time: 1 hour 10 minutes

14. Squash and Pear Soup

Ingredients:

- 1 medium butternut squash, peeled, seeded, and cubed
- 2 ripe pears, peeled, cored, and chopped
- 1 medium onion, chopped
- 2 cloves garlic, minced
- 4 cups low-sodium vegetable broth
- 1 cup almond milk (unsweetened)
- 1 tablespoon olive oil
- 1 teaspoon ground cinnamon
- 1/2 teaspoon ground nutmeg

Instructions:

1. In a large pot, heat the olive oil over medium heat. Add the onion and garlic, cooking until softened, about 5 minutes.
2. Add the cubed squash, chopped pears, vegetable broth, ground cinnamon, and ground nutmeg. Bring to a boil.
3. Reduce the heat and simmer for 20-25 minutes, or until the squash and pears are tender.
4. Use an immersion blender to puree the soup until smooth, or transfer to a blender in batches and blend until smooth.
5. Stir in the almond milk and heat through.
6. Serve warm.

Nutrition Info per Serving:

- Calories: 180
- Protein: 3g
- Carbohydrates: 35g
- Fat: 5g
- Fiber: 6g
- Sugar: 18g

Number of Serves: 4
Cooking Time: 30 minutes

15. Spinach and Potato Soup

Ingredients:

- 4 medium potatoes, peeled and cubed
- 1 medium onion, chopped
- 2 cloves garlic, minced
- 4 cups low-sodium vegetable broth
- 2 cups fresh spinach, chopped
- 1 cup almond milk (unsweetened)
- 1 tablespoon olive oil
- 1 teaspoon dried thyme

Instructions:

1. In a large pot, heat the olive oil over medium heat. Add the onion and garlic, cooking until softened, about 5 minutes.
2. Add the cubed potatoes, vegetable broth, and dried thyme. Bring to a boil.
3. Reduce the heat and simmer for 20-25 minutes, or until the potatoes are tender.
4. Use an immersion blender to puree the soup until smooth, or transfer to a blender in batches and blend until smooth.
5. Stir in the chopped spinach and almond milk. Cook for an additional 5 minutes, or until the spinach is wilted and the soup is heated through.
6. Serve warm.

Nutrition Info per Serving:

- Calories: 220
- Protein: 5g
- Carbohydrates: 40g
- Fat: 6g
- Fiber: 6g
- Sugar: 5g

Number of Serves: 4
Cooking Time: 30 minutes

16. Chicken Tortilla Soup

Ingredients:

- 1 lb (450g) boneless, skinless chicken breasts, cubed
- 1 medium onion, chopped
- 2 cloves garlic, minced
- 1 red bell pepper, chopped
- 1 cup corn kernels (fresh or frozen)
- 1 can (14.5 oz) diced tomatoes, no salt added
- 4 cups low-sodium chicken broth
- 1 tablespoon olive oil
- 1 teaspoon ground cumin
- 1 teaspoon dried oregano
- 1 teaspoon chili powder
- 4 corn tortillas, cut into strips
- 1 avocado, diced (optional)
- 1/4 cup fresh cilantro, chopped (optional)
- 1 lime, cut into wedges (optional)

Instructions:

1. In a large pot, heat the olive oil over medium heat. Add the onion, garlic, and red bell pepper, cooking until softened, about 5 minutes.
2. Add the cubed chicken and cook until browned on all sides.
3. Stir in the ground cumin, dried oregano, and chili powder, cooking for 1 minute.
4. Add the corn, diced tomatoes, and chicken broth. Bring to a boil, then reduce the heat and simmer for 20 minutes.
5. In a separate skillet, lightly toast the tortilla strips over medium heat until crisp, about 5 minutes.
6. Serve the soup topped with tortilla strips, diced avocado, fresh cilantro, and lime wedges if desired.

Nutrition Info per Serving:

- Calories: 320
- Protein: 28g
- Carbohydrates: 35g
- Fat: 10g
- Fiber: 6g
- Sugar: 6g

Number of Serves: 4
Cooking Time: 30 minutes

17. Lebanese Lentil Soup

Ingredients:

- 1 cup green or brown lentils, rinsed
- 1 medium onion, chopped
- 2 cloves garlic, minced
- 2 carrots, diced
- 2 celery stalks, diced
- 4 cups low-sodium vegetable broth
- 2 cups water
- 1 tablespoon olive oil
- 1 teaspoon ground cumin
- 1 teaspoon ground coriander
- 1/2 teaspoon ground turmeric
- 1/4 cup fresh lemon juice

Instructions:

1. In a large pot, heat the olive oil over medium heat. Add the onion, garlic, carrots, and celery, cooking until softened, about 5 minutes.
2. Stir in the ground cumin, ground coriander, and ground turmeric, cooking for 1 minute.
3. Add the lentils, vegetable broth, and water. Bring to a boil, then reduce the heat and simmer for 30-35 minutes, or until the lentils are tender.
4. Stir in the fresh lemon juice and cook for an additional 5 minutes.
5. Serve warm.

Nutrition Info per Serving:

- Calories: 220
- Protein: 10g
- Carbohydrates: 35g
- Fat: 5g
- Fiber: 12g
- Sugar: 5g

Number of Serves: 4
Cooking Time: 40 minutes

18. Zucchini Soup

Ingredients:

- 4 medium zucchinis, chopped
- 1 medium onion, chopped
- 2 cloves garlic, minced
- 4 cups low-sodium vegetable broth
- 1 cup almond milk (unsweetened)
- 1 tablespoon olive oil
- 1 teaspoon dried thyme

Instructions:

1. In a large pot, heat the olive oil over medium heat. Add the onion and garlic, cooking until softened, about 5 minutes.
2. Add the chopped zucchinis, vegetable broth, and dried thyme. Bring to a boil.
3. Reduce the heat and simmer for 15-20 minutes, or until the zucchinis are tender.
4. Use an immersion blender to puree the soup until smooth, or transfer to a blender in batches and blend until smooth.
5. Stir in the almond milk and heat through.
6. Serve warm.

Nutrition Info per Serving:

- Calories: 120
- Protein: 3g
- Carbohydrates: 18g
- Fat: 6g
- Fiber: 3g
- Sugar: 6g

Number of Serves: 4
Cooking Time: 25 minutes

19. Kale and White Bean Soup

Ingredients:

- 1 can (15 oz) white beans, rinsed and drained
- 4 cups kale, chopped
- 1 medium onion, chopped
- 2 cloves garlic, minced
- 4 cups low-sodium vegetable broth
- 2 cups water
- 2 carrots, sliced
- 2 celery stalks, sliced
- 1 tablespoon olive oil
- 1 teaspoon dried thyme
- 1/2 teaspoon dried rosemary

Instructions:

1. In a large pot, heat the olive oil over medium heat. Add the onion, garlic, carrots, and celery, cooking until softened, about 5 minutes.
2. Add the white beans, chopped kale, vegetable broth, water, dried thyme, and dried rosemary. Bring to a boil.
3. Reduce the heat and simmer for 20-25 minutes, or until the vegetables are tender.
4. Serve warm.

Nutrition Info per Serving:

- Calories: 180
- Protein: 8g
- Carbohydrates: 30g
- Fat: 4g
- Fiber: 8g
- Sugar: 5g

Number of Serves: 4
Cooking Time: 30 minutes

20. Moroccan Chickpea Stew

Ingredients:

- 1 can (15 oz) chickpeas, rinsed and drained
- 1 medium onion, chopped
- 2 cloves garlic, minced
- 2 carrots, diced
- 1 red bell pepper, chopped
- 1 can (14.5 oz) diced tomatoes, no salt added
- 4 cups low-sodium vegetable broth
- 1 tablespoon olive oil
- 1 teaspoon ground cumin
- 1 teaspoon ground cinnamon
- 1 teaspoon ground coriander
- 1/2 teaspoon ground ginger
- 1/4 cup fresh cilantro, chopped (optional)

Instructions:

1. In a large pot, heat the olive oil over medium heat. Add the onion, garlic, carrots, and red bell pepper, cooking until softened, about 5 minutes.
2. Stir in the ground cumin, ground cinnamon, ground coriander, and ground ginger, cooking for 1 minute.
3. Add the chickpeas, diced tomatoes, and vegetable broth. Bring to a boil, then reduce the heat and simmer for 20-25 minutes, or until the vegetables are tender.
4. Stir in the fresh cilantro, if using, just before serving.
5. Serve warm.

Nutrition Info per Serving:

- Calories: 200
- Protein: 8g
- Carbohydrates: 35g
- Fat: 5g
- Fiber: 8g
- Sugar: 10g

Number of Serves: 4
Cooking Time: 30 minutes

Snacks & Desserts

1. Banana and Peanut Butter Roll-Ups

Ingredients:

- 2 whole wheat tortillas
- 2 bananas, peeled
- 4 tablespoons natural peanut butter
- 1 tablespoon honey (optional)

Instructions:

1. Spread 2 tablespoons of peanut butter evenly over each whole wheat tortilla.
2. Place a banana in the center of each tortilla.
3. Drizzle honey over the bananas (optional).
4. Roll up the tortillas tightly around the bananas.
5. Slice each roll-up into bite-sized pieces and serve.

Nutrition Info per Serving:

- Calories: 250 Protein: 7g Carbohydrates: 40g Fat: 8g Fiber: 6g
- Sugar: 14g

Number of Serves: 2
Cooking Time: 5 minutes

2. Avocado Mousse

Ingredients:

- 2 ripe avocados, peeled and pitted
- 1/4 cup unsweetened cocoa powder
- 1/4 cup honey
- 1/2 cup almond milk (unsweetened)
- 1 teaspoon vanilla extract

Instructions:

1. In a blender or food processor, combine the avocados, cocoa powder, honey, almond milk, and vanilla extract.
2. Blend until smooth and creamy.
3. Spoon the mousse into serving bowls and refrigerate for at least 1 hour before serving.

Nutrition Info per Serving:

- Calories: 220 Protein: 3g Carbohydrates: 28g Fat: 13g
- Fiber: 7g
- Sugar: 19g

Number of Serves: 4
Cooking Time: 10 minutes (plus 1 hour refrigeration)

3. Smoothie Popsicles

Ingredients:

- 2 cups mixed berries (fresh or frozen)
- 1 banana, sliced
- 1 cup almond milk (unsweetened)
- 1 tablespoon honey (optional)

Instructions:

1. In a blender, combine the mixed berries, banana, almond milk, and honey (if using).
2. Blend until smooth.
3. Pour the mixture into popsicle molds and insert sticks.
4. Freeze for at least 4 hours, or until solid.
5. To serve, run warm water over the outside of the molds to release the popsicles.

Nutrition Info per Serving:

- Calories: 80
- Protein: 1g
- Carbohydrates: 19g
- Fat: 1g
- Fiber: 4g
- Sugar: 13g

Number of Serves: 6

Cooking Time: 10 minutes (plus 4 hours freezing)

4. Mashed Potato Cups

Ingredients:

- 4 medium potatoes, peeled and cubed
- 1/2 cup almond milk (unsweetened)
- 1/4 cup plain Greek yogurt
- 1 tablespoon olive oil
- 1 teaspoon dried thyme

Instructions:

1. Preheat the oven to 375°F (190°C).
2. In a large pot, boil the potatoes until tender, about 15 minutes. Drain and mash with the almond milk, Greek yogurt, olive oil, and dried thyme.
3. Spoon the mashed potatoes into a greased muffin tin, filling each cup about three-quarters full.
4. Bake for 20-25 minutes, or until the tops are lightly golden.
5. Allow to cool slightly before removing from the muffin tin and serving.

Nutrition Info per Serving:

- Calories: 100
- Protein: 2g
- Carbohydrates: 20g
- Fat: 2g
- Fiber: 2g
- Sugar: 2g

Number of Serves: 6
Cooking Time: 40 minutes

5. Soft Roasted Chickpeas

Ingredients:

- 1 can (15 oz) chickpeas, rinsed and drained
- 1 tablespoon olive oil
- 1 teaspoon ground cumin
- 1 teaspoon paprika
- 1/2 teaspoon garlic powder

Instructions:

1. Preheat the oven to 400°F (200°C).
2. In a bowl, toss the chickpeas with olive oil, ground cumin, paprika, and garlic powder until well coated.
3. Spread the chickpeas in a single layer on a baking sheet.
4. Bake for 20-25 minutes, or until the chickpeas are golden and slightly crispy.
5. Allow to cool slightly before serving.

Nutrition Info per Serving:

- Calories: 140
- Protein: 6g
- Carbohydrates: 20g
- Fat: 4g
- Fiber: 6g
- Sugar: 1g

Number of Serves: 4
Cooking Time: 30 minutes

6. Mini Cheese and Fruit Kabobs

Ingredients:

- 1 cup cheddar cheese, cubed
- 1 cup grapes
- 1 cup strawberries, hulled and halved
- 1 cup pineapple chunks
- 12 small wooden skewers

Instructions:

1. Thread one piece of cheddar cheese, one grape, one strawberry half, and one pineapple chunk onto each skewer.
2. Repeat until all ingredients are used.
3. Arrange the kabobs on a platter and serve immediately.

Nutrition Info per Serving:

- Calories: 100 Protein: 5g Carbohydrates: 12g Fat: 4g
- Fiber: 1g Sugar: 8g

Number of Serves: 6
Cooking Time: 10 minutes

7. Pumpkin Seed Trail Mix

Ingredients:

- 1 cup pumpkin seeds
- 1/2 cup almonds
- 1/2 cup dried cranberries
- 1/2 cup sunflower seeds
- 1/2 cup raisins

Instructions:

1. In a large bowl, combine the pumpkin seeds, almonds, dried cranberries, sunflower seeds, and raisins.
2. Mix well and store in an airtight container.
3. Serve as a snack.

Nutrition Info per Serving:

- Calories: 200
- Protein: 6g
- Carbohydrates: 24g
- Fat: 10g
- Fiber: 3g
- Sugar: 15g

Number of Serves: 6
Cooking Time: 5 minutes

8. Steamed Edamame

Ingredients:

- 2 cups edamame (fresh or frozen)
- 1 tablespoon low-sodium soy sauce
- 1 teaspoon sesame seeds (optional)

Instructions:

1. In a large pot, bring water to a boil. Add the edamame and cook for 3-5 minutes, or until tender.
2. Drain the edamame and transfer to a serving bowl.
3. Drizzle with low-sodium soy sauce and sprinkle with sesame seeds if using.
4. Serve warm.

Nutrition Info per Serving:

- Calories: 120
- Protein: 10g
- Carbohydrates: 10g
- Fat: 5g
- Fiber: 4g
- Sugar: 2g

Number of Serves: 4
Cooking Time: 10 minutes

9. Banana Cream Pie

Ingredients:

- **For the Crust:**
  - 1 1/2 cups graham cracker crumbs
  - 1/4 cup unsalted butter, melted
- For the Filling:
  - 3 ripe bananas, sliced
  - 1 package (3.4 oz) instant vanilla pudding mix
  - 2 cups almond milk (unsweetened)
  - 1 cup whipped cream (optional)

Instructions:

1. Preheat the oven to 350°F (175°C).
2. In a bowl, mix the graham cracker crumbs with melted butter until well combined. Press the mixture into the bottom of a 9-inch pie dish.
3. Bake the crust for 10 minutes. Remove from the oven and let it cool completely.
4. In a large bowl, whisk the instant vanilla pudding mix with almond milk until smooth. Refrigerate for 5 minutes to set.
5. Arrange the sliced bananas evenly over the cooled crust. Pour the pudding over the bananas, spreading it evenly.
6. Refrigerate the pie for at least 2 hours before serving. Top with whipped cream if desired.
7. Serve chilled.

Nutrition Info per Serving:

- Calories: 250
- Protein: 4g
- Carbohydrates: 40g
- Fat: 10g
- Fiber: 2g
- Sugar: 22g

Number of Serves: 8

Cooking Time: 20 minutes (plus refrigeration time)

10. Poached Pears in Vanilla Syrup

Ingredients:

- 4 ripe pears, peeled and cored
- 4 cups water
- 1 cup honey
- 1 vanilla bean, split and seeds scraped
- 1 tablespoon lemon juice

Instructions:

1. In a large pot, combine the water, honey, vanilla bean and seeds, and lemon juice. Bring to a simmer over medium heat.
2. Add the pears to the pot and simmer for 15-20 minutes, or until the pears are tender.
3. Remove the pears from the pot and let them cool slightly.
4. Continue to simmer the syrup for an additional 10 minutes, or until it thickens slightly.
5. Pour the syrup over the poached pears and refrigerate for at least 1 hour before serving.
6. Serve chilled.

Nutrition Info per Serving:

- Calories: 150
- Protein: 1g
- Carbohydrates: 38g
- Fat: 0g
- Fiber: 4g
- Sugar: 34g

Number of Serves: 4

Cooking Time: 30 minutes (plus refrigeration time)

11. Blueberry Yogurt Parfait

Ingredients:

- 2 cups plain Greek yogurt
- 1 cup fresh blueberries
- 1/2 cup granola
- 2 tablespoons honey
- 1 teaspoon vanilla extract

Instructions:

1. In a bowl, mix the Greek yogurt, honey, and vanilla extract until well combined.
2. In serving glasses or bowls, layer the Greek yogurt mixture, fresh blueberries, and granola.
3. Repeat the layers until all ingredients are used.
4. Serve immediately or refrigerate until ready to serve.

Nutrition Info per Serving:

- Calories: 180
- Protein: 10g
- Carbohydrates: 28g
- Fat: 5g
- Fiber: 3g
- Sugar: 20g

Number of Serves: 4

Cooking Time: 10 minutes

12. Pumpkin Custard

Ingredients:

- 1 cup pumpkin puree
- 1 cup almond milk (unsweetened)
- 2 large eggs
- 1/4 cup honey
- 1 teaspoon ground cinnamon
- 1/2 teaspoon ground nutmeg
- 1/2 teaspoon ground ginger

Instructions:

1. Preheat the oven to 350°F (175°C).
2. In a large bowl, whisk together the pumpkin puree, almond milk, eggs, honey, ground cinnamon, ground nutmeg, and ground ginger until smooth.
3. Pour the mixture into individual custard cups or ramekins.
4. Place the custard cups in a baking dish and fill the dish with hot water until it reaches halfway up the sides of the cups.
5. Bake for 30-35 minutes, or until the custards are set.
6. Remove from the oven and let cool. Refrigerate for at least 2 hours before serving.

Nutrition Info per Serving:

- Calories: 120
- Protein: 5g
- Carbohydrates: 18g
- Fat: 4g
- Fiber: 2g
- Sugar: 15g

Number of Serves: 4

Cooking Time: 40 minutes (plus refrigeration time)

13. Vanilla Panna Cotta

Ingredients:

- 1 cup almond milk (unsweetened)
- 1 cup plain Greek yogurt
- 1/4 cup honey
- 1 teaspoon vanilla extract
- 1 packet (2.5 tsp) unflavored gelatin
- 2 tablespoons cold water

Instructions:

1. In a small bowl, sprinkle the gelatin over the cold water and let it sit for 5 minutes to bloom.
2. In a saucepan, heat the almond milk and honey over medium heat until just warm (do not boil).
3. Remove from heat and stir in the bloomed gelatin until fully dissolved.
4. Whisk in the Greek yogurt and vanilla extract until smooth.
5. Pour the mixture into individual serving cups or ramekins.
6. Refrigerate for at least 4 hours, or until set.
7. Serve chilled, optionally topped with fresh berries or a fruit compote.

Nutrition Info per Serving:

- Calories: 120
- Protein: 6g
- Carbohydrates: 20g
- Fat: 2g
- Fiber: 0g
- Sugar: 18g

Number of Serves: 4

Cooking Time: 10 minutes (plus 4 hours refrigeration time)

10-WEEK MEAL PLAN

Week 1
Monday
- Breakfast: Barley Porridge with Dates and Almonds
- Lunch: Chicken Noodle Soup
- Snack: Soft Roasted Chickpeas
- Dinner: Balsamic Glazed Chicken

Tuesday
- Breakfast: Peach and Ginger Compote
- Lunch: Turkey and Sweet Potato Stew
- Snack: Mashed Potato Cups
- Dinner: Shrimp and Rice Pilaf

Wednesday
- Breakfast: Raspberry and Walnut Oatmeal
- Lunch: Lentil Soup with Spinach
- Snack: Avocado Mousse
- Dinner: Grilled Trout with Herbs

Thursday
- Breakfast: Egg Custard
- Lunch: Butternut Squash Soup
- Snack: Smoothie Popsicles
- Dinner: Cod in Papillote with Vegetables

Friday
- Breakfast: Kefir with Honey and Almonds
- Lunch: Chicken and Prune Tagine
- Snack: Mini Cheese and Fruit Kabobs
- Dinner: Lemon Tilapia with Herbed Quinoa

Saturday
- Breakfast: Soft French Toast with Apple Compote
- Lunch: Chicken Porridge with Vegetables
- Snack: Pumpkin Seed Trail Mix
- Dinner: Miso Glazed Cod

Sunday
- Breakfast: Chia Pudding with Kiwi
- Lunch: Sweet Potato and Coconut Milk Soup
- Snack: Steamed Edamame
- Dinner: Turkey Shepherd's Pie

Week 2

Monday
- Breakfast: Baked Sweet Potatoes with Yogurt and Chives
- Lunch: Tomato Basil Soup
- Snack: Blueberry Yogurt Parfait
- Dinner: Chicken Risotto

Tuesday
- Breakfast: Sweet Corn Cakes
- Lunch: Lebanese Lentil Soup
- Snack: Poached Pears in Vanilla Syrup
- Dinner: Salmon and Spinach Potato Casserole

Wednesday
- Breakfast: Steamed Vegetable Medley with Poached Eggs
- Lunch: Split Pea Soup with Ham
- Snack: Pumpkin Custard
- Dinner: Turkey and Butternut Squash Hash

Thursday
- Breakfast: Quinoa Breakfast Bowl
- Lunch: Carrot and Ginger Puree Soup
- Snack: Banana and Peanut Butter Roll-Ups
- Dinner: Shrimp Risotto

Friday
- Breakfast: Chicken Congee
- Lunch: Zucchini Soup
- Snack: Banana Cream Pie
- Dinner: Pan-Seared Tuna with Olive Tapenade

Saturday
- Breakfast: Peanut Butter Banana Smoothie
- Lunch: Kale and White Bean Soup
- Snack: Avocado Mousse
- Dinner: Baked Snapper with Tomato and Basil

Sunday
- Breakfast: Greek Yogurt Parfait
- Lunch: Creamy Butternut Squash Soup
- Snack: Soft Roasted Chickpeas
- Dinner: Turkey Piccata

Week 3

Monday
- Breakfast: Sweet Potato Hash with Soft Cooked Eggs
- Lunch: Cauliflower and Turmeric Soup
- Snack: Mini Cheese and Fruit Kabobs
- Dinner: Chicken Tortilla Soup

Tuesday
- Breakfast: Pumpkin Porridge
- Lunch: Moroccan Chickpea Stew
- Snack: Smoothie Popsicles
- Dinner: Seafood Pasta in White Sauce

Wednesday
- Breakfast: Mashed Potato Bowl with Scrambled Eggs
- Lunch: Potato Leek Soup
- Snack: Pumpkin Seed Trail Mix
- Dinner: Grilled Trout with Herbs

Thursday
- Breakfast: Spinach and Cheese Stuffed Crepes
- Lunch: Squash and Pear Soup
- Snack: Steamed Edamame
- Dinner: Chicken and Dumplings

Friday
- Breakfast: Butternut Squash Soup
- Lunch: Spinach and Potato Soup
- Snack: Poached Pears in Vanilla Syrup
- Dinner: Fish Pie with Mashed Potato Topping

Saturday
- Breakfast: Herbed Scrambled Tofu
- Lunch: Sweet Potato and Coconut Milk Soup
- Snack: Banana and Peanut Butter Roll-Ups
- Dinner: Turkey and Vegetable Loaf

Sunday
- Breakfast: Pancakes with Ricotta and Orange Zest
- Lunch: Lebanese Lentil Soup
- Snack: Avocado Mousse
- Dinner: Shrimp and Rice Pilaf

Week 4

Monday
- Breakfast: Vegetable Omelette
- Lunch: Split Pea Soup with Ham
- Snack: Mashed Potato Cups
- Dinner: Chicken Tortilla Soup

Tuesday
- Breakfast: Quinoa Breakfast Bowl
- Lunch: Carrot and Ginger Puree Soup
- Snack: Smoothie Popsicles
- Dinner: Turkey Shepherd's Pie

Wednesday
- Breakfast: Chicken Congee
- Lunch: Kale and White Bean Soup
- Snack: Banana Cream Pie
- Dinner: Pan-Seared Tuna with Olive Tapenade

Thursday
- Breakfast: Peanut Butter Banana Smoothie
- Lunch: Zucchini Soup
- Snack: Poached Pears in Vanilla Syrup
- Dinner: Baked Snapper with Tomato and Basil

Friday
- Breakfast: Greek Yogurt Parfait
- Lunch: Moroccan Chickpea Stew
- Snack: Soft Roasted Chickpeas
- Dinner: Grilled Trout with Herbs

Saturday
- Breakfast: Sweet Potato Hash with Soft Cooked Eggs
- Lunch: Potato Leek Soup
- Snack: Pumpkin Seed Trail Mix
- Dinner: Chicken and Prune Tagine

Sunday
- Breakfast: Pumpkin Porridge
- Lunch: Squash and Pear Soup
- Snack: Steamed Edamame
- Dinner: Fish Pie with Mashed Potato Topping

Week 5

Monday
- Breakfast: Mashed Potato Bowl with Scrambled Eggs
- Lunch: Spinach and Potato Soup
- Snack: Banana and Peanut Butter Roll-Ups
- Dinner: Turkey and Vegetable Loaf

Tuesday
- Breakfast: Spinach and Cheese Stuffed Crepes
- Lunch: Sweet Potato and Coconut Milk Soup
- Snack: Smoothie Popsicles
- Dinner: Grilled Trout with Herbs

Wednesday
- Breakfast: Herbed Scrambled Tofu
- Lunch: Moroccan Chickpea Stew
- Snack: Poached Pears in Vanilla Syrup
- Dinner: Seafood Pasta in White Sauce

Thursday
- Breakfast: Pancakes with Ricotta and Orange Zest
- Lunch: Kale and White Bean Soup
- Snack: Avocado Mousse
- Dinner: Shrimp and Rice Pilaf

Friday
- Breakfast: Vegetable Omelette
- Lunch: Split Pea Soup with Ham
- Snack: Mashed Potato Cups
- Dinner: Chicken Tortilla Soup

Saturday
- Breakfast: Quinoa Breakfast Bowl
- Lunch: Carrot and Ginger Puree Soup
- Snack: Smoothie Popsicles
- Dinner: Turkey Shepherd's Pie

Sunday
- Breakfast: Chicken Congee
- Lunch: Potato Leek Soup
- Snack: Pumpkin Seed Trail Mix
- Dinner: Baked Snapper with Tomato and BasiL

Week 6

Monday
- Breakfast: Banana and Peanut Butter Roll-Ups
- Lunch: Creamy Butternut Squash Soup
- Snack: Mini Cheese and Fruit Kabobs
- Dinner: Salmon Patties with Cucumber Yogurt Sauce

Tuesday
- Breakfast: Pumpkin Custard
- Lunch: Chicken Tortilla Soup
- Snack: Steamed Edamame
- Dinner: Pan-Seared Tuna with Olive Tapenade

Wednesday
- Breakfast: Avocado Mousse
- Lunch: Zucchini Soup
- Snack: Pumpkin Seed Trail Mix
- Dinner: Lemon Tilapia with Herbed Quinoa

Thursday
- Breakfast: Blueberry Yogurt Parfait
- Lunch: Split Pea Soup with Ham
- Snack: Soft Roasted Chickpeas
- Dinner: Balsamic Glazed Chicken

Friday
- Breakfast: Smoothie Popsicles
- Lunch: Moroccan Chickpea Stew
- Snack: Poached Pears in Vanilla Syrup
- Dinner: Grilled Trout with Herbs

Saturday
- Breakfast: Mashed Potato Cups
- Lunch: Sweet Potato and Coconut Milk Soup
- Snack: Banana Cream Pie
- Dinner: Cod in Papillote with Vegetables

Sunday
- Breakfast: Greek Yogurt Parfait
- Lunch: Cauliflower and Turmeric Soup
- Snack: Mini Cheese and Fruit Kabobs
- Dinner: Chicken and Dumplings

Week 7

Monday
- Breakfast: Quinoa Breakfast Bowl
- Lunch: Tomato Basil Soup
- Snack: Avocado Mousse
- Dinner: Turkey and Sweet Potato Stew

Tuesday
- Breakfast: Peanut Butter Banana Smoothie
- Lunch: Split Pea Soup with Ham
- Snack: Pumpkin Seed Trail Mix
- Dinner: Baked Salmon with Spinach and Potatoes

Wednesday
- Breakfast: Blueberry Yogurt Parfait
- Lunch: Carrot and Ginger Puree Soup
- Snack: Soft Roasted Chickpeas
- Dinner: Shrimp Fried Rice

Thursday
- Breakfast: Mashed Potato Bowl with Scrambled Eggs
- Lunch: Chicken Tortilla Soup
- Snack: Steamed Edamame
- Dinner: Grilled Trout with Herbs

Friday
- Breakfast: Pumpkin Custard
- Lunch: Sweet Potato and Coconut Milk Soup
- Snack: Banana and Peanut Butter Roll-Ups
- Dinner: Fish Pie with Mashed Potato Topping

Saturday
- Breakfast: Avocado Mousse
- Lunch: Zucchini Soup
- Snack: Poached Pears in Vanilla Syrup
- Dinner: Seafood Pasta in White Sauce

Sunday
- Breakfast: Smoothie Popsicles
- Lunch: Moroccan Chickpea Stew
- Snack: Mashed Potato Cups
- Dinner: Pan-Seared Tuna with Olive Tapenade

Week 8

Monday
- Breakfast: Greek Yogurt Parfait
- Lunch: Kale and White Bean Soup
- Snack: Soft Roasted Chickpeas
- Dinner: Lemon Tilapia with Herbed Quinoa

Tuesday
- Breakfast: Banana and Peanut Butter Roll-Ups
- Lunch: Tomato Basil Soup
- Snack: Mini Cheese and Fruit Kabobs
- Dinner: Grilled Salmon with Lemon and Dill

Wednesday
- Breakfast: Blueberry Yogurt Parfait
- Lunch: Chicken Porridge with Vegetables
- Snack: Steamed Edamame
- Dinner: Cod in Papillote with Vegetables

Thursday
- Breakfast: Pumpkin Custard
- Lunch: Cauliflower and Turmeric Soup
- Snack: Smoothie Popsicles
- Dinner: Turkey and Butternut Squash Hash

Friday
- Breakfast: Peanut Butter Banana Smoothie
- Lunch: Split Pea Soup with Ham
- Snack: Banana Cream Pie
- Dinner: Baked Snapper with Tomato and Basil

Saturday
- Breakfast: Avocado Mousse
- Lunch: Moroccan Chickpea Stew
- Snack: Soft Roasted Chickpeas
- Dinner: Pan-Seared Tuna with Olive Tapenade

Sunday
- Breakfast: Quinoa Breakfast Bowl
- Lunch: Sweet Potato and Coconut Milk Soup
- Snack: Mashed Potato Cups
- Dinner: Grilled Trout with Herbs

Week 9
Monday
- Breakfast: Greek Yogurt Parfait
- Lunch: Tomato Basil Soup
- Snack: Poached Pears in Vanilla Syrup
- Dinner: Salmon and Spinach Potato Casserole

Tuesday
- Breakfast: Banana and Peanut Butter Roll-Ups
- Lunch: Chicken Tortilla Soup
- Snack: Smoothie Popsicles
- Dinner: Turkey and Sweet Potato Stew

Wednesday
- Breakfast: Blueberry Yogurt Parfait
- Lunch: Zucchini Soup
- Snack: Steamed Edamame
- Dinner: Balsamic Glazed Chicken

Thursday
- Breakfast: Pumpkin Custard
- Lunch: Sweet Potato and Coconut Milk Soup
- Snack: Mashed Potato Cups
- Dinner: Grilled Salmon with Lemon and Dill

Friday
- Breakfast: Peanut Butter Banana Smoothie
- Lunch: Moroccan Chickpea Stew
- Snack: Soft Roasted Chickpeas
- Dinner: Pan-Seared Tuna with Olive Tapenade

Saturday
- Breakfast: Avocado Mousse
- Lunch: Cauliflower and Turmeric Soup
- Snack: Mini Cheese and Fruit Kabobs
- Dinner: Seafood Pasta in White Sauce

Sunday
- Breakfast: Quinoa Breakfast Bowl
- Lunch: Kale and White Bean Soup
- Snack: Banana Cream Pie
- Dinner: Cod in Papillote with Vegetables

WEEKLY MEAL PLANNER + WORKBOOK

	BREAKFAST	LUNCH	DINNER	SNACKS
MONDAY				
TUESDAY				
WEDNESDAY				
THURSDAY				
FRIDAY				
SATURDAY				
SUNDAY				

Describe your typical daily meals and snacks before undergoing chemotherapy. What were your go-to foods and beverages?

....

....

....

....

....

....

WEEKLY MEAL PLANNER + WORKBOOK

	BREAKFAST	LUNCH	DINNER	SNACKS
MONDAY				
TUESDAY				
WEDNESDAY				
THURSDAY				
FRIDAY				
SATURDAY				
SUNDAY				

Reflect on your favorite indulgences or comfort foods before chemotherapy. How do you plan to satisfy these cravings while following a chemo diet?

....

....

....

....

....

....

WEEKLY MEAL PLANNER + WORKBOOK

	BREAKFAST	LUNCH	DINNER	SNACKS
MONDAY				
TUESDAY				
WEDNESDAY				
THURSDAY				
FRIDAY				
SATURDAY				
SUNDAY				

List any dietary habits or patterns you had before chemotherapy that you believe may need to change or adjust during treatment. Why are these changes necessary?

....

....

....

....

....

....

WEEKLY MEAL PLANNER + WORKBOOK

	BREAKFAST	LUNCH	DINNER	SNACKS
MONDAY				
TUESDAY				
WEDNESDAY				
THURSDAY				
FRIDAY				
SATURDAY				
SUNDAY				

Think about your hydration habits before chemotherapy. How did you ensure you stayed hydrated, and how will you continue to prioritize hydration during treatment?

....

....

....

....

....

....

WEEKLY MEAL PLANNER + WORKBOOK

	BREAKFAST	LUNCH	DINNER	SNACKS
MONDAY				
TUESDAY				
WEDNESDAY				
THURSDAY				
FRIDAY				
SATURDAY				
SUNDAY				

What are your main concerns or challenges about starting a chemo diet? How do you plan to address these challenges?

....

....

....

....

....

....

WEEKLY MEAL PLANNER + WORKBOOK

	BREAKFAST	LUNCH	DINNER	SNACKS
MONDAY				
TUESDAY				
WEDNESDAY				
THURSDAY				
FRIDAY				
SATURDAY				
SUNDAY				

Identify three new foods or ingredients you're willing to incorporate into your diet to support your recovery. What benefits do you expect from including these items?

....

....

....

....

....

....

WEEKLY MEAL PLANNER + WORKBOOK

	BREAKFAST	LUNCH	DINNER	SNACKS
MONDAY				
TUESDAY				
WEDNESDAY				
THURSDAY				
FRIDAY				
SATURDAY				
SUNDAY				

Reflect on any changes in appetite or taste preferences since starting chemotherapy. How will you adapt your meals to accommodate these changes?

....

....

....

....

....

....

WEEKLY MEAL PLANNER + WORKBOOK

	BREAKFAST	LUNCH	DINNER	SNACKS
MONDAY				
TUESDAY				
WEDNESDAY				
THURSDAY				
FRIDAY				
SATURDAY				
SUNDAY				

Consider your support system. How can family and friends assist you in maintaining a chemo diet and overall wellness during treatment?

....

....

....

....

....

....

WEEKLY MEAL PLANNER + WORKBOOK

	BREAKFAST	LUNCH	DINNER	SNACKS
MONDAY				
TUESDAY				
WEDNESDAY				
THURSDAY				
FRIDAY				
SATURDAY				
SUNDAY				

Reflect on any digestive issues or gastrointestinal symptoms you've experienced since starting chemotherapy. How do you plan to manage these through your diet?

....

....

....

....

....

....

WEEKLY MEAL PLANNER + WORKBOOK

	BREAKFAST	LUNCH	DINNER	SNACKS
MONDAY				
TUESDAY				
WEDNESDAY				
THURSDAY				
FRIDAY				
SATURDAY				
SUNDAY				

Reflect on your goals for following a chemo diet. How do you plan to measure success and adjust your approach based on your progress and experiences?

....

....

....

....

....

WEEKLY MEAL PLANNER + WORKBOOK

	BREAKFAST	LUNCH	DINNER	SNACKS
MONDAY				
TUESDAY				
WEDNESDAY				
THURSDAY				
FRIDAY				
SATURDAY				
SUNDAY				

What are your expectations regarding energy levels and overall well-being as you transition to a chemo diet?

....

....

....

....

....

....

WEEKLY MEAL PLANNER + WORKBOOK

	BREAKFAST	LUNCH	DINNER	SNACKS
MONDAY				
TUESDAY				
WEDNESDAY				
THURSDAY				
FRIDAY				
SATURDAY				
SUNDAY				

Consider any dietary restrictions or guidelines provided by your healthcare team. How do these recommendations influence your meal planning and food choices?

....

....

....

....

....

....

Scan the QR code below to get a surprise bonus!

Made in the USA
Columbia, SC
05 December 2024

48532200R00078